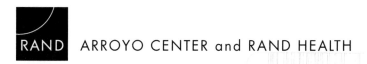

RAND ARROYO CENTER and RAND HEALTH

T0108967

Patient Privacy, Consent, and Identity Management in Health Information Exchange

Issues for the Military Health System

Susan D. Hosek, Susan G. Straus

Prepared for the United States Army

The research described in this report was sponsored by the United States Army Medical Research and Materiel Command, Telemedicine and Advanced Technology Research Center (TATRC). It was conducted jointly by RAND Health and RAND Arroyo Center, a federally funded research and development center for the U.S. Army.

Library of Congress Cataloging-in-Publication Data

Hosek, Susan D.
  Patient privacy, consent, and identity management in health information exchange : issues for the military health system / Susan D. Hosek, Susan G. Straus.
    pages cm
  Includes bibliographical references.
  ISBN 978-0-8330-7790-5 (pbk. : alk. paper)
  1. Medical records—Access control—United States. 2. United States—Armed Forces—Medical care. 3. Medicine, Military—United States—Information services. 4. Medical informatics—United States. 5. Information storage and retrieval systems—Medical care. I. Straus, Susan G. II. Title.

  R864.H67 2013
  610.285—dc23   2013015711

The RAND Corporation is a nonprofit institution that helps improve policy and decisionmaking through research and analysis. RAND's publications do not necessarily reflect the opinions of its research clients and sponsors.

RAND® is a registered trademark.

Published 2013 by the RAND Corporation
1776 Main Street, P.O. Box 2138, Santa Monica, CA 90407-2138
1200 South Hayes Street, Arlington, VA 22202-5050
4570 Fifth Avenue, Suite 600, Pittsburgh, PA 15213-2665
RAND URL: http://www.rand.org/
To order RAND documents or to obtain additional information, contact
Distribution Services: Telephone: (310) 451-7002;
Fax: (310) 451-6915; Email: order@rand.org

Preface

This report presents findings for a project entitled "Policy Issues for Health Information Technology and Health Informatics," for which RAND was asked to analyze policy issues related to the development of a research initiative on health information technology and health informatics within the Department of Defense's (DoD's) Military Health System (MHS). The project was in support of a Joint Program Committee-1b (JPC-1b) effort to develop a roadmap for the research initiative.

RAND was asked to focus on policy, research findings, and experiences with respect to patient privacy, consent, and identity management as relevant to health information exchange (HIE). The report focuses specifically on HIE between DoD, the Department of Veterans Affairs (VA), and civilian health care providers who treat the departments' beneficiaries. In addition to policymakers involved in managing health information technology and health information exchange in DoD and VA, the report should be of interest to audiences interested in health information exchange for a large, nationally distributed patient population.

The U.S. Army Medical Research and Materiel Command, Telemedicine and Advanced Technology Research Center (TATRC), sponsored this study. It was conducted jointly by RAND Health and the RAND Arroyo Center, a federally funded research and development center for the U.S. Army.

The Project Unique Identification Code (PUIC) for the project that produced this document is HQD116051.

Contents

Figure

Tables

Summary

The Military Health System (MHS) and the Veterans Health Administration (VHA) have been among the nation's leaders in health information technology (IT), including the development of health IT systems and electronic health records (EHRs) that summarize patients' care from multiple providers. Health IT interoperability within MHS and across MHS partners, including VHA, is one of ten goals in the current MHS Strategic Plan; the ability to exchange health information between military and nonmilitary health care providers is especially important in light of the role played by civilian providers in MHS's TRICARE program, which provides care to 9.7 million beneficiaries.

The MHS has taken several steps toward achieving improved interoperability, including collaborating with the Department of Veterans Affairs (VA) to develop an integrated EHR, a virtual lifetime electronic record (VLER), and Joint Federal Health Care Centers. The MHS is also seeking to develop a research roadmap to better coordinate health IT research efforts, address MHS IT capability gaps, and reduce programmatic risk for enterprise projects in the MHS. This report contributes to that effort by identifying key research and policy issues involving patient privacy, patient consent, and patient identity management as relevant to health information exchange (HIE) in the Department of Defense (DoD). Our study used a multimethod approach consisting of a review of policy regarding privacy, patient consent, and patient identity management; a literature review on these topics as relevant to the MHS; and semistructured telephone interviews with 31 subject-matter experts. We use a sociotechnical framework to organize our findings and to suggest topics for future research.

Privacy of Individual Health Information

The shift from paper medical records to electronic records raises new concerns about privacy, the protection of which is key to patient consent and identity matching.

Legislation and Policy

The federal government mandated the protection of protected health information (PHI) by health care organizations 16 years ago, through the Health Insurance Portability and Accountability Act of 1996 (HIPAA). HIPAA established federal standards designed to safeguard individual health records while allowing for the exchange of information to ensure the quality of health care and public health. The HIPAA Privacy Rule regulates the disclosure and use of individuals' PHI that is or has been maintained or transmitted electronically by covered health care entities. Some states have copied the HIPAA provisions into state law, sometimes adding restrictions on the disclosure of PHI relating to especially sensitive areas such as mental health or the human immunodeficiency virus (HIV).

The Department of Health and Human Services (DHHS) has developed a framework identifying privacy protection and information security principles that health information organizations (HIOs) should follow. Among the principles outlined are individuals' right to access their information through simple and timely means; the right to dispute the accuracy or integrity of their information and correct it or have their dispute recorded; and the need for transparency about policies, procedures, and technologies that affect patients or their PHI. Similar frameworks have been developed by other public and private health care organizations.

Considerations for DoD and VA Concerning Privacy

There is widespread consensus on the principles that should guide HIE, including the need for consent for HIE and accuracy in linking EHR information to patients. However, there is less consensus about the specific approaches used to implement these principles. The goal of policy is to design approaches that find the right balance between the beneficial use of EHRs and privacy protection.

Patient Consent

Patient consent or authorization for HIE is central to the issue of privacy, yet there is often ambiguity and controversy about the meaning of *consent* and the mechanisms for obtaining it. For example, responses to requests for public comment on the proposed HIPAA rule revealed that many individuals felt that they "own" their health records and should be asked for permission to release PHI for every request. Nonetheless, survey data indicate that a large majority of Americans support HIE to improve health care.

Consent Regulations

There are a number of federal regulations governing consent requirements for use and disclosure of PHI. The HIPAA Privacy Rule attempts to create a balance between safeguarding individuals' privacy and allowing for the disclosure and use of information to promote health care quality and efficiency. There are several situations or activities, including treatment, payment, or health care operations, for which covered entities can disclose PHI without first obtaining authorization from patients. Patients must be allowed to request restrictions on the disclosure of their information for permitted uses, but covered entities are not required to agree to these requests. Other federal regulations pertaining to consent for HIE govern the disclosure of clinical laboratory results, substance abuse treatment program records, and records of treatment for drug abuse, alcohol abuse or alcoholism, infection with HIV/AIDs, and sickle cell anemia by the VHA.

There are also myriad state laws regarding disclosure of PHI. The central issue with respect to patient consent is that electronic transmission facilitates the exchange of information across states, yet states have different disclosure requirements. Providers accessing information on a patient from another state must adhere to the disclosure requirements of that state, which are likely to differ from and may conflict with the requirements in their state.

Consent Principles

Valid, informed consent consists of five elements: disclosure, capacity or competence, understanding or comprehension, voluntariness, and consent or decision. There are also multiple models of patient consent, ranging from *no consent*, in which HIE occurs automatically (which applies to active duty personnel), to various *opt-out* (in which HIE occurs by default) and *opt-in* (in which HIE requires written authorization) models. Most health exchange initiatives use opt-out consent at the provider or organizational level, and while both opt-in and opt-out consent can be implemented poorly, it is more difficult to ensure disclosure, capacity, and understanding for all patients using an opt-out approach. As a result, opt-out approaches may not reflect voluntary decisionmaking on the part of patients.

Recently, approaches to obtaining patient consent have tended to shift control of the process from providers to patients. Patient- or person-centric approaches, in which each patient is given a unique identifier and then accesses a single location to specify their preferences for HIE nationwide, offer numerous benefits, but also pose challenges. Centralized consent offers consumers control over who gets their PHI, for what purposes, and over what time frame. The approach also eliminates the need for providers to maintain separate records of patients' consent preferences. However, consumer-centric approaches require providers to have the means to store and access the consent service ID in their systems, and successful adoption depends on a variety of sociotechnical factors, including patients' willingness to manage their own consent data. If a patient puts restrictions on the content of the health information that can be exchanged, the provider's system must be capable of granular HIE (which limits data access and use based on factors such as the recipient, purpose, duration, and content of patient health information) or the provider must be willing to filter the patient's data manually.

Considerations for DoD and the VA Regarding Patient Consent

We anticipate that a number of changes in mechanisms for consent will be needed to support the VLER:

- DoD will need the capacity to record and implement patients' restrictions on the disclosure of PHI when they are approved under the current opt-out procedure.
- Retaining PHI from non-DoD providers will require implementing any disclosure restrictions on secondary disclosure. Current methods for granular consent are in their infancy.
- Research on the design and usability of automated text processing to redact restricted patient information, particularly in unstructured data such as clinical notes, is needed.

We expect that it may be difficult to proceed with VLER without a meaningful consent procedure that reflects the principles proposed by the Office of the National Coordinator for Health Information Technology's HIT Policy Committee "Tiger Team" (which call for "meaningful, revocable" consent for HIE other than direct provider-to-provider exchange). Although HIPAA allows providers to share patient health information for treatment, payment, and operations without patient authorization, we expect that many civilian providers may not be able or willing to do so. DoD may conclude that the best approach is to follow the VA in developing a patient consent management system for non–active duty beneficiaries.

To be meaningful, the consent procedure must adequately inform patients about the choices they have and the consequences of those choices, and the procedure must be conducted in a manner that ensures that consent is entirely voluntary. If DoD determines that there should be some kind of consent for HIE through VLER, research is needed to guide decisions about the type of consent, beneficiary outreach and education, and the procedure(s) to be followed.

Proactive research, carried out in the unique context of the military, would inform the development of future consent policy and the design of next-generation health IT systems. Additional topics for a research agenda on patient consent would include:

- pilot tests of patient consent management systems in clinical settings to assess their uptake and effectiveness
- analyzing and designing workflows to administer informed consent; ensuring that it is meaningful or valid in terms of disclosure, capacity, understanding, and voluntariness; and verifying consent for HIE at the point of care.

Patient Identity Management

Key issues involved in patient identity management include the identifiers to be used to link individual patients to their PHI and the approach used to identify an individual patient across multiple health care organizations.

Choice of Identifiers
PHI can be linked to individual patients through a number of identifiers, such as name, address, email address, phone number, or a unique patient identifying number (e.g., Social Security number [SSN]). Non-unique, out-of-date, or incorrect identifiers can lead to errors, including false negatives (failure to find a patient's information when it in fact exists) and false positives (finding information that is not, in fact, the patient's).

Identity Matching
Identity matching is the process used to identify the same individual across health care organizations using the specified identifiers for HIE. Numerous methods are available, from simple deterministic algorithms that require an exact match on the specified identifiers to highly sophisticated probabilistic, hierarchical algorithms in which a threshold must be set to establish a match.

Patient Matching Approach
Together, the choice of identifiers and a matching algorithm constitute a patient matching approach. Often, deciding which approach to use

means trading off between the false positive and false negative rates. Approaches that have a very low probability of matching to the wrong person also often lead to an increase in false negatives—not successfully matching to information available from other providers. Maximizing the successful match rate often comes at a cost of increasing the false positive rate—linking to the wrong patient information. Unique and accurate patient identifiers can lower both types of errors, as can more effective matching algorithms.

Without a national system of unique patient identifiers, patient identity matching for HIE poses difficult challenges. Even if a unique patient identifier were established, the potential for errors in recording it would require additional matching on other patient identifiers to ensure that the right patient's information is being exchanged. Considering the different combinations of patient identifiers that are potentially available and the many algorithms that can be adapted to this use, the number of patient identity matching approaches is very large.

Although studies have examined the different outcomes of matching approaches based on types of identifiers and matching algorithms, none of the research has been conducted in a functioning HIO with multiple providers. The studies use either simulated or proxy patient indexes and researchers instead of HIO managers to implement the matching algorithms. Thus, the literature provides very limited real-world information on which to base a choice of patient identifiers, matching algorithm, match criteria, and manual review of the results of automated matching.

Considerations for DoD and VA Regarding Patient Identity Management

More research is needed to assess the cost-effectiveness of the different options in practice, using actual patient registries or electronic medical records and the business processes that providers and HIOs are likely to sustain over time. DoD and VA could inform their own choices and contribute valuable information to guide others through investigation of the performance of promising approaches for nationwide implementation of VLER for all beneficiaries, including military family members:

- The research should evaluate to the maximum extent possible the performance of different approaches in matching at the scale that will be required for VLER at the national level once more civilian providers participate in the MHS's health network.
    - The research should use actual identifying data from the Person Data Repository, test performance at scale, and pilot promising approaches in the clinical setting.
    - The research should measure the trade-offs among key performance technical outcomes, including time needed to complete a patient information request, false negative and positive rates, and the expertise and resources needed for development and maintenance of the matching approach.
- A parallel line of research should focus on other issues related to implementation within organizations, such as work processes at the facility and system levels for ensuring the accuracy of patient identifying information, procedures at the clinical level that increase the efficient retrieval of electronic information from other providers to support patient care, and best practices for checking that the information received is for the right patient and is accurate.

As with patient consent, there are policy issues to resolve within organizations and at the federal and state levels regarding the type of identifiers that can maintain patient privacy.

Finally, following a sociotechnical approach, it is important to consider how technical, social, and organizational factors work together. Addressing isolated issues regarding patient identity management and consent will not be productive; research and implementation needs to address multiple factors and their interactions in supporting successful HIE.

Acknowledgements

We would like to thank Steve Steffensen (Chief Medical Information Officer), Ollie Gray, Betty Levine, and Bob Connors at TATRC for their assistance and guidance throughout this project.

We conducted numerous interviews during this study, and we are indebted to those in the military health community who shared their time and expertise.

We also wish to thank RAND colleagues who contributed to this effort. Edward Chan participated in many of the interviews for this study and provided background material for several topics. Danielle Meeker provided material on granular consent for Chapter Three and advice throughout the project. Spencer Jones, Bob Rudin, and Geoffrey McGovern contributed helpful information at the beginning of this effort. Kristin Leuschner drafted the summary of this monograph. We received valuable suggestions that helped us improve the report from our technical reviewers, Tora Bikson and Linda Dimitropolous.

Abbreviations

ARRA	American Recovery and Reinvestment Act
CCD	continuity of care document
CDC	Centers for Disease Control and Prevention
CFR	Code of Federal Regulations
CLIA	Clinical Laboratory Improvement Amendment
CMS	Centers for Medicare and Medicaid Services
DBN	DoD Benefits Number
DHHS	Department of Health and Human Services
DMDC	Defense Manpower Data Center
DoD	Department of Defense
EDI-PI	Electronic Data Interchange Personal Identifier
EHR	electronic health record
FTE	full-time equivalent
HIE	health information exchange
HIMSS	Healthcare Information and Management Systems Society
HIO	health information organization

HIPAA	Health Insurance Portability and Accountability Act
HITECH	Health Information Technology for Economic and Clinical Health Act
HITSP	Healthcare Information Technology Standards Panel
HIV	human immunodeficiency virus
HMO	health maintenance organization
iEHR	integrated electronic health record
IOM	Institute of Medicine
IT	information technology
JPC-1b	Joint Program Committee-1b on Health Information Technology and Medical Informatics
MAeHC	Massachusetts eHealth Collaborative
MHS	Military Health System
MTF	military treatment facility
NLP	natural language processing
NwHIN	Nationwide Health Information Network
ONC	Office of the National Coordinator for Health Information Technology
PDR	Person Data Repository
PHI	protected health information
PHR	personal health record
PPO	preferred provider organization
RHIO	regional health information organization
RLS	record-locator service

SCR	summary care record
SSA	Social Security Administration
SSN	Social Security number
TATRC	Telemedicine and Advanced Technology Research Center
TMA	TRICARE Management Activity
VA	Department of Veterans Affairs
VHA	Veterans Health Administration
VLER	virtual lifetime electronic record

CHAPTER ONE
Introduction and Background

The Military Health System (MHS) and the Veterans Health Administration (VHA) have been among the nation's leaders in health information technology (IT). They have been leaders in the development of health IT systems and electronic health records (EHRs) that summarize patients' care from multiple providers.[1] Since the Gulf War and during the conflicts in Iraq and Afghanistan, there has been renewed interest in the coordination of health care activities in the Department of Defense (DoD) and Department of Veterans Affairs (VA), including the sharing of capabilities to improve health care cost effectiveness, to better understand combat-related health risks, and to smoothly transition health care responsibility and information for service members when they become veterans (President's Task Force to Improve Health Care Delivery for the Nation's Veterans, 2003; President's Commission on Care for America's Returning Wounded Warriors, 2007).

Health IT interoperability within MHS and across MHS partners, including VHA, is one of ten goals in the current MHS Strategic Plan. MHS plans to achieve this goal by (1) collaborating with the VA to develop an integrated EHR, a virtual lifetime electronic record (VLER), and Joint Federal Health Care Centers; (2) establishing interoperability with other business partners, including private sector health care organizations, by developing policies, business rules, and

[1] The Healthcare Information and Management Systems Society (HIMSS) (2006) distinguishes between an electronic medical record, which is the detailed record of care delivered by a provider organization, and an EHR, which is a summary of care delivered by multiple provider organizations.

1

information exchange services; (3) achieving technical and semantic interoperability to enable a common view of data; and (4) defining an integration strategy with initiatives by the Department of Health and Human Services' (DHHS's) Office of the National Coordinator for Health Information Technology (ONC) to encourage adoption of health IT and health information exchange (HIE) nationally.

The MHS has established a Joint Program Committee on Health Information Technology and Medical Informatics (JPC-1b) with members from the Telemedicine and Advanced Technology Research Center (TATRC), Office of the Secretary of Defense, the Joint Staff, and the services to provide funding recommendations and program management support for research on health IT. Contributing to this effort is the development of a research roadmap that is intended to better coordinate health IT research efforts, address current MHS IT capability gaps through well-focused research initiatives, and reduce programmatic risk for enterprise projects in the MHS. The roadmap will guide the selection of research initiatives, provide a foundation or baseline by which to evaluate the adoption of innovative health IT systems and services, assist in the coordination of research initiatives, and facilitate the transfer of results from those initiatives to the enterprise IT organizations within the MHS.

RAND was asked to contribute information for roadmap development on patient privacy, consent, and identity management as relevant to HIE in the DoD. For each topic, the objectives were to identify (1) relevant policy, (2) findings from the research literature, and (3) user experiences. The remainder of this section provides an overview of our study approach, background on the MHS and its initiatives for HIE with the VA and civilian providers, the current status of HIE in the United States, and a framework for organizing the issues we address.

Study Approach

To meet our study objectives, we used a multimethod approach consisting of (1) a review of policy regarding patient privacy, consent, and identity management; (2) a search and review of research literature on these topics as relevant to the MHS; and (3) semistructured telephone interviews with 31 subject-matter experts from a variety of organizations and with diverse responsibilities and expertise. Interview participants included key staff and stakeholders from

- TRICARE Management Activity (TMA)
- Defense Manpower Data Center (DMDC)
- service personnel involved with DoD-VA HIE pilots
- TATRC contractors working on relevant health IT research
- a patient privacy rights organization.

One to three RAND researchers conducted each of the interviews. Questions were adapted to the responsibilities of each organization and interviewee. For VLER pilot sites and other services engaged in health care delivery, we addressed the organization's current approach to patient privacy, consent, and identity management; the extent to which the organization collects data by testing the effectiveness of their practices (e.g., match rates or consent rates); and anticipated changes in approaches and procedures. Interviews with other stakeholders addressed policy or research related to privacy, consent, and identity management. In all interviews, we discussed obstacles and lessons learned regarding the focal topics. Findings and recommendations are organized using a sociotechnical systems framework, as described later in this chapter and in the concluding chapter of this report.

Military Health System

Through its TRICARE program, DoD's MHS provides care to 9.7 million beneficiaries, including active duty personnel, activated Guard/Reserve personnel, military retirees, eligible family members, and survivors.[2] Almost half of this care is provided directly in military treatment facilities (MTFs)—56 military hospitals and 365 ambulatory care clinics. The remainder of the care is provided through an extensive

---

[2]   Data and other information from TRICARE (2012).

network of civilian providers who contract with TRICARE—3,224 hospitals, 438,424 individual providers, and 64,712 retail pharmacies—and military medical units supporting operations in Afghanistan, Iraq, and elsewhere.

TRICARE includes two enrollment options for beneficiaries under age 65: a health maintenance organization (HMO) called TRICARE Prime and a preferred provider organization (PPO) called TRICARE Standard/Extra.[3] Active duty personnel (including activated Guard/Reserve personnel) are automatically enrolled in the HMO, and other beneficiaries have a choice. At age 65, beneficiaries shift their primary coverage to Medicare, and the TRICARE for Life program supplements Medicare. TRICARE also includes smaller programs for non-activated Guard/Reserve personnel interested in purchasing TRICARE coverage for themselves and their family members. HMO enrollment totaled 5.5 million in 2011; 83.5 percent of all beneficiaries used some TRICARE services.

MHS Goals and Initiatives

Health care costs have been increasing rapidly, and the fiscal year 2012 budget for TRICARE, $54 billion, is expected to account for 7 percent of the DoD budget. At the same time, a paramount MHS mission is to maintain the medical readiness of military personnel and to care for the wartime wounded and other service members whose health is affected by their military service. The MHS has established the MHS Quadruple Aim—four goals to guide management of the system (Table 1.1).

To pursue these four goals, the MHS is implementing the patient-centered medical home concept in military primary-care clinics. These clinics primarily serve active duty personnel and beneficiaries who are enrolled in TRICARE Prime and assigned for primary care to an MTF. Under this concept, MTF primary care managers are accountable for integrating all primary, specialty, and ancillary care for an assigned

---

[3] The Extra option in the PPO is limited to services provided by a network provider, whereas the Standard option covers care from a non-network provider. Provider payment rates and patient cost sharing differ for network and non-network care.

Table 1.1
MHS Quadruple Aim

Goal	Description
Readiness	Ensure that military personnel are medically ready to deploy and that the MHS is ready to deliver health care in support of military operations
Population health	Encourage healthy behaviors and decrease the population illness rate through prevention
Experience of care	Provide care that is patient- and family-centered, compassionate, convenient, equitable, safe, and always of the highest quality
Per capita cost	Manage health care costs over time by focusing on quality, eliminating waste, and reducing unwarranted variation

SOURCE: TRICARE (2012).

enrollee panel, including care provided by other military providers and through referral to the civilian network. Performance is regularly monitored through metrics tracking access to care and to the primary care managers in particular, utilization of services, cost, quality, patient and provider satisfaction, and medical readiness.

Electronic Health Record

Information management and information technology for the MHS is guided by a five-year strategic plan. The plan identifies the importance of providing timely access to information to meet the objectives identified in the Quadruple Aim and establishes a priority of developing a "robust EHR . . . [that will] be intuitive, aggregate data for each patient over time and across providers, operate in all care settings, and allow sharing of information with our health partners" (Military Health System, 2009, p. 9). The benefits of health IT in a military environment are substantial, but the MHS also poses some unique challenges to implementation. Military commanders need timely access to health information for assessing the medical readiness of the personnel they command. Military providers must have worldwide access to their patients' health records in MTFs and a wide range of field environments. Even in peacetime, military personnel (and their families) move to new assignments about every three years, as do military providers. Over the past decade, top priority has been given to ensuring that providers treating the war wounded in theater medical units, MTFs, and the VA have the information they need to provide the best possible care.

The MHS recognized the value of an EHR early and began developing health IT systems in the 1980s. Currently it has an EHR covering care provided in MTFs and a comprehensive pharmacy system. Purchased civilian care is captured through the claims submitted for reimbursement. A third-generation EHR is in the early stages of development in collaboration with the VA through a joint-department Integrated Program Office. One important goal of moving to an integrated EHR (iEHR) with the VA is to facilitate the exchange of health information for military personnel and veterans who are using or have used both MHS and VA services and to support other sharing arrangements between the two departments, including joint medical facilities serving both military and veteran populations with a mix of DoD and VA medical staff.

In light of the important role of civilian providers in caring for TRICARE beneficiaries, the ability to exchange health information with these providers will be critical to the success of the patient-centered medical home. MTFs vary widely in size and medical capability. Although some MTFs support a range of medical specialties and subspecialties, many are limited to primary care and perhaps some degree of specialty care. Enrollees at these MTFs receive their specialty care in the community, and their primary care managers can do little without extensive access to information regarding the patients' health care histories and referral care. In our discussions with DoD officials, the importance of HIE with civilian providers came up frequently.

Virtual Lifetime Electronic Record

After separation from military service, veterans (including retirees) may continue to get health care and benefits from DoD, but they are also eligible for VA benefits, including health care, disability benefits, education benefits (e.g., the GI Bill), and employment services. During their period of service, some military personnel also get health care through the VA. To confirm eligibility and transfer the information needed to provide these various benefits, DoD and the VA have set up a number of information-sharing arrangements over time. The VLER is intended to systematize and expand these arrangements in an integrated information system capturing health, benefits, and administrative information beginning with accession into military service. The information resides in many locations, but the VLER system provides authorized users with on-demand access to the information.

VLER will be implemented in phases, with each phase expanding the information available to users (Department of Defense and Department of Veterans Affairs, 2011). The first stage will provide the capability to exchange summary of care and certain clinical documents between DoD, the VA, and civilian providers treating service members and veterans.[4] The goals are to (1) improve the flow of information for referrals, dual DoD-VA system users, and individuals who also receive care through other insurance, including Medicare, Medicaid, and employer coverage and (2) enhance clinical decision support. VLER relies on ONC's Nationwide Health Information Network (NwHIN), which is a set of standards, services, and policies to enable secure HIE over the Internet, and the direct exchange of information between DoD and the VA where possible either currently or when the iEHR will be implemented.

DoD and the VA have been piloting VLER in a number of locations where there is an integrated health care organization or regional health information organization (RHIO) participating in NwHIN. The first pilot was established in the winter of 2009 in San Diego with the San Diego VA Medical Center, Naval Medical Center San Diego, and Kaiser Permanente. Kaiser is not a TRICARE network provider, so opportunities to share information for military patients at this site have been limited. Currently, VA has ten pilot sites, including four co-located with an MTF (Figure 1.1). A decision will be made in summer

---

[4] Later phases will support exchange of more comprehensive health information, including that needed for adjudicating VA disability claims and enhanced computability as data standards and technology permit.

2012 about implementing VLER nationwide for DoD and VA and in all locations where there are or could be civilian participants in NwHIN.

The three VLER sites involving DoD as an active participant are

- Tidewater, Virginia (fall 2010): Naval Medical Center Portsmouth, Hampton VA Medical Center, Med Virginia
- Spokane, Washington (spring 2011): 92nd Medical Group at Fairchild Air Force Base, Spokane VA Medical Center, Inland Northwest Health Services (INHS)
- Puget Sound, Washington (fall 2011): Madigan Army Medical Center, Puget Sound VA Health Care System, MultiCare.

The MTFs in the Tidewater and Puget Sound areas are among the largest medical centers in the MHS and home to specialty residency training programs. They are a major referral source for TRI-CARE beneficiaries in all TRICARE plans. In contrast, the MTF in

Figure 1.1
VLER Pilot Sites

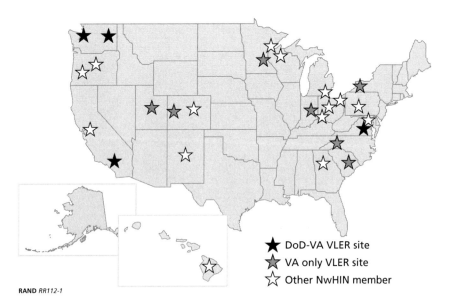

Spokane is a primary care clinic and must refer its patients to civilian providers for specialty care.

In these VLER pilots, the MTFs exchange information for their active duty and retired patients who also receive care from another VLER participant. Information for family members is not being exchanged in the pilots.

We interviewed the person responsible for VLER at each of these sites and several individuals involved in the project at TMA and DMDC. The information we gathered about the pilots' experiences with VLER is incorporated in subsequent sections of this report.

DoD and the VA have committed to a decision on national roll-out in summer 2012 (*Interagency Program Office: Annual Report to Congress*, 2011). Although the departments are committed to implementing VLER, the limited number of civilian providers participating in NwHIN will restrict areas where HIE can be expanded to include civilian providers. Further, DoD has not yet made a decision about when and how to expand VLER to include all beneficiaries.

Health Information Exchange in the United States

Health Information Organizations

A health information organization (HIO) or health information exchange organization is "An organization that oversees and governs the exchange of health-related information among organizations according to nationally recognized standards" (National Alliance for Health Information Technology, 2008). Multiple models of access to patients' data for HIE within HIOs have been identified (HIMSS, 2012; Wilcox et al., 2006). They differ in where patient data are stored and how providers access the information. A centralized model collects patient data from providers and stores them in a centralized data repository. Requests for patient information are directed to the central repository. The more common federated model retains patient data in the data repositories of the individual entities providing care and facilitates authorized access to the information by other providers through a record-locator service (RLS) typically maintained by an HIO. The

RLS is an index that indicates only whether health information for patients exists among participating organizations. The RLS contains patient identifying information (e.g., name, birth date) and indicates the organizations in which the patient has had care. A provider seeking clinical information about a patient queries the RLS to identify where the patient has received care; the provider can then request data from those organizations and must comply with the disclosure requirements of each organization. Thus, in a federated model, providers maintain control over their patients' data. Other models combine features of centralized and federated models, for example by storing patient data in a centralized repository with provider-specific directories, or by giving patients control over their data.

Promoting Adoption of Health Information Technology and Health Information Exchange

The federal government is promoting adoption of EHRs and HIE through a number of initiatives. In 2004, the ONC was established within DHHS by executive order. ONC has a wide range of development, implementation, and research programs intended to support nationwide adoption of health IT. NwHIN, the Direct Project, and CONNECT software are of particular relevance to this report.[5]

- As noted earlier, NwHIN (formerly NHIN) enables secure HIE over the Internet via standards, services, and policies. Although NwHIN was initially referred to as a network of networks, according to ONC, NwHIN is not a physical network that supports HIE. The NwHIN-Exchange is an association of public and private entities that are exchanging patient health information consisting of summary records for care coordination (including the VLER), summary records for Social Security Administration (SSA) disability determination, and bio-surveillance and case reporting to the Centers for Disease Control and Prevention (CDC). As of March 2012, NwHIN-Exchange had 27 participants, including four federal agencies (Centers for Medicare and

---

[5] See The Office of the National Coordinator for Health Information Technology, 2011.

Medicaid Services [CMS], DoD, VA, and SSA), local and state HIOs, and other networks.

- The Direct Project is developing standards and services to enable secure, directed electronic HIE at a more local level, such as a primary care provider sending a referral or care summary to a local specialist. The Direct Project is complementary to NwHIN.
- CONNECT is open-source software that supports HIE using national standards for interoperability.

ONC also coordinates the programs to implement the Health Information Technology for Economic and Clinical Health Act (HITECH), which was enacted in 2009 as part of the American Recovery and Reinvestment Act (ARRA). HITECH directed the government to take a leadership role in developing standards for nationwide HIE, expanded on the privacy and security requirements of the Health Insurance Portability and Accountability Act of 1996 (HIPAA) (discussed later in this report), and set forth criteria and incentives for "meaningful use" of EHRs. Meaningful use criteria are intended to motivate not only the adoption but also the use of EHRs that bring about significant improvements in health care quality, safety, and efficiency; reduced health disparities; increased patient/family engagement; better care coordination; and improved population and public health. EHR users are expected to achieve these outcomes while maintaining privacy and security. Eligible professionals and hospitals that can demonstrate meaningful use of certified EHRs may qualify for CMS incentive payments under the Medicare and Medicaid EHR Incentive Programs. Beginning in 2015, eligible Medicare providers who do not adopt a certified EHR will be subject to penalties in the form of reduced Medicare payments. Certification ensures that users can achieve meaningful use criteria and that data are secure, confidential, and can be shared with other systems. ONC determined the criteria and process by which EHR systems are certified.

HITECH specifies three stages of meaningful use of a certified EHR, with the expectation that, in Stages 2 and 3, providers will meet the criteria of previous stages, including those criteria that were optional.

- Stage 1 focuses on data capture and sharing, i.e., using capabilities of EHRs that capture health information in a structured format. To qualify for incentives, hospitals and eligible professionals must demonstrate compliance with a core set of objectives, such as using computerized provider order entry, clinical summaries, and drug-drug and drug-allergy interaction checks and maintaining up-to-date problem lists; as well as compliance with five of ten menu objectives, such as implementing drug-formulary checks and incorporating clinical lab-test results into the EHR as structured data. The final rule (42 CFR Parts 412, 413, 422, and 495) was published on July 28, 2010, and Stage 1 began in calendar year 2011.
- Stage 2 focuses on the use of health IT for quality improvement at the point of care and on electronic exchange of health information. Thus, HIE is a primary goal of Stage 2 meaningful use, with the aim of moving providers toward full HIE. CMS issued the proposed rule for Stage 2 criteria in March 2012. It includes changes to some Stage 1 criteria and proposes a one-year delay for Stage 2 (to 2014) so that providers can accommodate needed changes in technology and workflow.
- Stage 3 focuses on improvements in quality, safety, and efficiency; use of clinical decision support; access to patient self-management tools; access to comprehensive patient data through patient-centered health information exchange; and improving population health. Stage 3 is scheduled to begin in 2016.

Status of Health Information Exchange

Two recent studies have evaluated the state of HIE in the U.S. The first study, by Adler-Milstein, Bates, and Jha (2011), focused on RHIOs, which have a number of advantages over separate agreements for HIE in terms of mission, technical infrastructure, cost, and community support. Adler-Milstein, Bates, and Jha surveyed all 197 potential RHIOs in the United States. Of 165 RHIOs that completed the survey, 75 (46 percent), comprising approximately 14 percent of U.S. hospitals and 3 percent of ambulatory practices, actively facilitated clinical data exchange between independent entities. Although the number of RHIOs had increased over previous years' surveys, only 13 RHIOs, comprising 3 percent of hospitals and 0.9 percent of ambulatory practices, supported the types of data exchange required under Stage 1 meaningful use, and only 6 of the 75 operational RHIOs (8 percent) met both the core and optional Stage 1 meaningful use criteria. None of the RHIOs met subject-matter experts' criteria for comprehensive HIE. Finally, only 33 percent of the operational RHIOs reported being financially viable. Thus, although several aspects of RHIOs may be particularly conducive to HIE, the authors questioned whether RHIOs in their current form can support the data exchange needed to attain anticipated improvements in quality and efficiency of care.

The second study, by the eHealth Initiative (2011), surveyed communities across the United States with initiatives to share health information. This study covered a broader range of health exchange initiatives than RHIOs, including academic institutions, community-based nonprofit and for-profit organizations, hospital-based or integrated delivery networks, Medicaid agencies, and public health agencies. In comparison to the 2009 and 2010 results, the study showed large increases in the numbers of initiatives meeting Stage 1 meaningful use criteria as well as modest increases in those meeting proposed Stage 2 criteria. Of the 196 communities included in the study, only 24 reported that they were self-sustaining (up from 18 in 2010).[6] These communities continued to deal with issues affecting the privacy and confidentiality of the information being exchanged and with challenges in technical architecture and performance.

Frameworks for Evaluating Health Information Technology

A number of authors have proposed frameworks for evaluating health IT adoption and effectiveness. A common theme in the literature, as well as in research on organizations more generally, is that there are a number of interrelated factors that contribute to successful change in organizations. Many studies of IT adoption use a sociotechnical

---

[6] These results are not directly comparable to Adler-Milstein, Bates, and Jha (2011) because the nature of health exchange initiatives was different in the studies.

approach, which emphasizes the importance of the social and organizational context in combination with technical factors in fostering uptake of IT (Davis, Bagozzi, and Warshaw, 1989; Venkatesh and Davis, 2000; Venkatesh et al., 2003). According to the Institute of Medicine (IOM) (2012), health IT ". . . encompasses a technical system of computers and software that operates in the context of a larger sociotechnical system—a collection of hardware and software working in concert within an organization that includes people, processes, and technology" (pp. S-1 to S-2).

Examples of sociotechnical frameworks applied to health IT adoption and effectiveness are those proposed by Creekmore, Piescik, and Gershon (2010), Sicotte and Paré (2010), Sittig and Singh (2007), and the IOM (2012). These frameworks are similar in content but vary somewhat in how constructs are labeled and organized (for example, some models group hardware and software by usability issues, whereas other models treat them separately) and, in some cases, constructs are defined more or less broadly. Creekmore, Piescik, and Gershon[7] identified eight contextual facilitators and barriers to large-scale change, which they grouped into four quadrants: external context, policy context, structural context, and behavioral context. Sicotte and Paré's framework consists of five dimensions of risk: technological, human, usability, managerial, and political. Sittig and Singh identified eight dimensions in their model: hardware and software computing infrastructure; clinical content; human-computer interface; people; workflow and communication; internal organizational policies, procedures, and culture; external rules, regulations, and pressures; and system measurement and monitoring.

Any of these frameworks can be useful as a way to think about the design, development, implementation, and evaluation of health IT systems. We have selected the IOM (2012) framework, which was used in a recent report on health IT and patient safety, as an organizing tool, as we find it parsimoniously reflects facilitators and challenges to health IT issues in MHS. The report delineates five components of any sociotechnical system and describes their relevance to health IT safety:

---

[7]   Cited from West and Friedman (2012).

- *Technology*, i.e., hardware and software.
- *People*, i.e., the individuals who use the system. This component includes individuals' knowledge and skills with respect to technology and clinical work.
- *Process*, or the actions and procedures that clinicians are expected to perform when delivering health care. Process is often referred to as workflow.
- *Organization* refers to ". . . how the organization installs health IT, makes configuration choices, and specifies interfaces with health IT products" (IOM, 2012, pp. 3–4). It includes strategic goals (such as a patient safety culture) and rules and regulations.
- *External environment* is the environment in which organizations operate, especially with regard to regulations of federal, state, and private sector entities with which health care organizations must comply.

In sociotechnical systems theory, the dimensions that comprise the system interact with each other. Thus, when planning to implement new technological systems or diagnose problems with existing systems, these factors must be considered in concert. Analyzing only one factor (e.g., attributing a problem to human error) or considering multiple factors without regard to their interrelationships is likely to lead to inaccurate diagnoses and inappropriate remedial strategies or plans.

Because our focus differs from the IOM's topic of analysis, we define the five dimensions somewhat more broadly, integrating some of the concepts from the other models. For example, in the "people" category, we include attitudes (Creekmore, Bagozzi, and Gershon, 2010; Sicotte and Paré, 2010) in addition to knowledge and skills, and we specify a range of stakeholders (Sittig and Singh, 2007) in addition to clinicians. Our definitions of the categories are shown in Table 1.2. We reference these constructs in our discussion of patient privacy, consent, and identity management, and we use the framework to identify issues, research gaps, and recommendations for future research in the concluding chapter of this report.

Table 1.2
IOM Health Information Technology Framework (Adapted)

Factor	Definition
Technical	Hardware and software, including access, design, development, and standards.
People	Individuals who develop, implement, use, and are affected by the system, which include IT staff, clinical staff, administrators, commanders, and patients. Encompasses attitudes, knowledge, and skills.
Process	Activities and procedures that people engage in when using the system.
Organization	(Internal) strategic goals, decisions, rules, regulations, and policies with respect to IT use and clinical practice. Includes resources available to support programs.
Environment	Policy environment in which organizations operate; include DoD, other federal agencies, states, and private sector entities.

Another underlying theme in our discussion is the notion of trade-offs. Health IT design and implementation decisions often involve striking a balance between different, and sometimes conflicting, goals. Examples include attaining maximum benefits of HIE for health care quality and maintaining patient privacy, and using automated approaches and minimizing error rates.

Organization of This Report

Chapter Two sets the context for our analysis by presenting an overview of privacy issues, policy, and public attitudes related to HIE. Privacy has been a long-standing concern in handling patient information, long before the arrival of health IT, and it plays a central role in health policy via HIPAA. Chapters Three and Four address two key topics in the privacy domain: patient consent and patient identity management, respectively. For each topic, we review (1) background (e.g., definitions) and existing policy; (2) potential approaches for handling each function; and (3) research findings and experiences in practice.

The final chapter concludes with a summary of findings and identified research gaps organized by the framework presented above.

CHAPTER TWO

Privacy of Individual Health Information

The shift from paper medical records to electronic records raises new concerns about privacy. Access to paper records for individual patients is limited to authorized personnel at the treating provider organization, including providers, clinical support staff, and administrative personnel. The same personnel may also access individual patients' electronic records. However, unlike paper records, electronic records can be disclosed in very large numbers, for example, through inadvertent loss or theft of computer storage devices. As more protected health information (PHI) is made available to networks of providers, the business associates of providers, and for secondary uses such as research and marketing, the risk of disclosure increases. With paper records, patients can be fairly certain that they know where their records are located and that only a limited number of people will see their information at this location. With increasing electronic storage, sharing, and use of PHI, patients cannot be certain of who has their information, how it is being used, or how well protected it is from inadvertent disclosure or security breaches.

Concerns about the privacy of PHI have been prominent in the policy debate regarding the federal role in health IT. A major report by the President's Council of Advisors on Science and Technology (2010) identified legitimate patient concerns about privacy and security as one of four major barriers to the development of effective health IT systems. It concluded:

> Innate, strong, privacy protection on all data, both at rest and
> in transit, with persistent patient-controlled privacy preferences,
> is . . . achievable, and must be designed in from the start. (p. 4)

The report identified four factors leading to concern about the privacy of medical data: (1) discrimination in health insurance coverage and employment based on health status, (2) exploitive use of the data for commercial interests, (3) the desire to keep government agencies from accessing private information, and (4) the unique nature of health information and the common desire to keep it private. Press reports of inadvertent disclosure of health records and other sensitive information draw public attention to the privacy risk associated with the growing adoption of health IT.

As we discuss below, the federal government mandated protection of PHI by health care organizations 16 years ago, before the widespread availability of health IT systems that enable providers to exchange electronic records. Growing awareness of the potential for health IT to improve the cost-effectiveness of health care has led to federal and state initiatives to promote adoption and to ensure appropriate access to and use of the information. Inadequately addressed privacy concerns could pose a barrier to adoption if providers and patients withhold information that would contribute to better care or lower costs. Therefore, the goal of policy is to design approaches that find a good balance between the beneficial use of electronic health records and privacy protection.

In this section, we review the requirements in the law for privacy protection in the United States, public opinion on issues related to the privacy of PHI, and frameworks laying out principles that should govern HIE. Privacy is a priority for all aspects of electronic health information collection, storage, and disclosure. In the succeeding chapters, we describe the important role privacy plays in designing policies and approaches related to patient consent and identity management.

Legal Requirements

HIPAA established standards for protecting health information (Office for Civil Rights, 2003). The standards were designed to safeguard individual health records while allowing for the exchange of information to ensure the quality of health care and public health. The requirements laid out in HIPAA were implemented by DHHS in the Privacy Rule.[1] The Privacy Rule applies to all health plans that provide or pay for health care; providers exchanging information for referrals to other providers, health care claims, business operations, or other specified purposes; health care clearinghouses; and certain business associates of covered entities. The HIPAA protections apply to health information in which the individual is identified directly or may be identifiable by inference, usually referred to as PHI. The rule permits disclosure for (1) treatment, payment, and health care operations and (2) a number of public-interest purposes, including specified government, law enforcement, and public health activities; military operations; and research. Disclosure for these purposes does not require patient consent, but disclosure for some other purposes does require consent. Patients may request access to and correction of their PHI and an audit trail of disclosures. They also may request restrictions on disclosure for the uses permitted under HIPAA, and, if an entity agrees to the restrictions, it is responsible for implementing the restrictions. Finally, HIPAA directed DHHS to develop standards for establishing unique national identifiers for health providers, health plans, and patients. Concerns about privacy protection led Congress to withhold funding for developing the unique patient identifier system until the technology for ensuring the protection of health information is in place.

When HIPAA was enacted, health IT was in the earliest stage of development. More recently, recognizing the potential for health IT systems to improve the cost-effectiveness of care, Congress passed HITECH,[2] which strengthened the HIPAA privacy protections in sev-

---

[1]   45 CFR Part 160 and Subparts A and E of Part 164.

[2]   Title XIII of Division A and Title IV of Division B of the American Recovery and Reinvestment Act (ARRA) of 2009 (Pub. L. 111–5).

eral ways. First, it expanded the definition of business associates to include organizations that routinely access and transmit PHI, such as RHIOs and HIOs, and it subjected business associates to the same security requirements and penalties as health plans and health care providers. Second, it specified requirements for notifying those individuals whose PHI has been breached. Third, it directed DHHS to provide education to covered entities and individuals about their rights and responsibilities regarding the privacy and security of PHI. Fourth, it directed DHSS to issue guidance on the definition of minimum necessary information and gave patients more rights regarding their data in electronic format. Fifth, it prohibited the sale of EHRs or PHI, with some exceptions. Finally, HITECH mandated stronger enforcement of federal PHI privacy regulations and established stronger penalties for violations.

At the federal level, additional privacy requirements are levied for records of care provided in substance abuse treatment programs and for treatment of drug abuse, alcoholism or alcohol abuse, and, in the VA, infection with the human immunodeficiency virus (HIV) or sickle cell anemia.[3] However, these requirements do not apply to the exchange of PHI between DoD and the VA. DoD regulation allows for the disclosure of protected PHI for military personnel by any covered entity when it is "deemed necessary by appropriate military command authorities to assure the proper execution of the military mission" or upon separation from military service to support determination of benefits eligibility.[4]

States vary in their laws governing the privacy of PHI. Some states have no provisions or have adopted the HIPAA provisions, but other states have added restrictions on disclosure of PHI relating to especially sensitive areas such as mental health or HIV. The state provisions are not applicable to care provided in MHS or VA facilities, but civilian providers may feel bound by them except when they treat active-duty patients.

---

[3]   42 CFR Part 2 and 38 CFR Part 1.

[4]   DoD 6025.18-R, Section C7.11.1

Researchers studying privacy and HIE have noted that federal privacy protections leave some gaps as information exchange capabilities grow, inhibiting trust in HIE (Greenberg, Ridgely, and Hillestad, 2009; McGraw et al., 2009). For example, network design characteristics and the oversight and accountability mechanisms have yet to be established and tested to ensure that PHI shared over a widely distributed network is appropriately protected once it leaves the control of the initial holder of the information. McGraw et al. (2009) also note the need for policy changes to strengthen privacy protections in HIPAA and instill trust in HIE; for example, by clearly defining health care operations, tightening restrictions on secondary uses of PHI for marketing purposes, and revisiting standards in the Privacy Rule to ensure that there is minimal risk of re-identifying de-identified data.[5]

Public Attitudes

In recent years, there have been a number of studies of public attitudes related to HIE benefits and privacy. The results consistently indicate that individuals also perceive the trade-off between the two, balancing belief in the potential for improving health care and outcomes with concern about privacy and security of their PHI in electronic systems capable of sharing data.

The Markle Survey on Health in a Networked Life (Markle Foundation, 2011) collected information about health care issues using the Knowledge Networks' nationally representative online survey panel. The survey was conducted on a sample of adults (1,582 respondents) and also a sample of physicians (779 respondents). Eighty percent of individual respondents and almost as many physicians agreed that physicians should be required to share PHI for the purpose of reducing errors, improving coordination of care, and avoiding duplication of medical services. The same percentage favored strong privacy protec-

---

[5] HIPAA allows covered entities to provide de-identified data to third parties for uses such as research or business planning. If the recipient re-identifies the data, which is relatively easy to accomplish in some cases, the re-identified data are not subject to HIPAA.

tions, including patients' rights regarding their information: notification of unauthorized access; a list of who has had access; a clear process to request corrections; and the ability to make informed choices about collection, use, and disclosure. Most respondents did not support government access to their identifiable information.

The California HealthCare Foundation commissioned a survey of a representative sample of 1,849 adults from the same Knowledge Networks panel in late 2009 and early 2010 (Westat, 2009). Many of the questions focused on use of and interest in personal health records (PHRs) but also included some more general questions about privacy and HIE that complement the Markle survey. When asked about potential barriers to using a PHR, three-quarters of respondents not using a PHR agreed that they worried about the privacy of their information. However, almost as many (61 percent) also indicated that they did not need a PHR to handle their health needs. More generally, 68 percent of all respondents were very or somewhat concerned about the privacy of their medical records, and only 31 percent were comfortable having their information shared with other organizations such as health plans, researchers, or companies.[6]

In a third survey, involving telephone interviews and a random-digit-dial sample, almost 70 percent of the 1,847 respondents reported that they were very or somewhat concerned about the privacy of HIE (Dimitropoulos et al., 2011). The percentage expressing concern was higher for respondents age 40 and above and, reflecting widespread concern about disclosure to employers, for those who were employed full-time. Two-thirds of respondents indicated that it was very or somewhat important to them to be able to restrict access to their information by providers not involved in their care, friends, employers, and payers. Only half as many expressed a desire to limit access to their providers and family.

As we describe in Chapter Four, there are privacy risks associated with identity management, e.g., linking health information to the

---

[6]   Rates of PHR use in other countries range from 5–7 percent in Canada, France, and Switzerland to 16 percent in Belgium and Brazil and 31 percent in China. Concern about risk is widespread; the U.S. results are in the mid-to-low range of the 12 countries in the survey.

wrong patient or not finding a patient's information. Dimitropoulos et al. included questions on this issue in their survey. A majority of the respondents thought that it was very or somewhat likely that their information would be linked to the wrong person or disclosed to the wrong provider.

Despite these concerns about privacy, surveys show strong consumer support for HIE. Almost 90 percent of the respondents to the Dimitropoulos et al. survey thought that HIE would improve coordination of care, and 75 percent thought it would improve quality of care.[7] Seventy-five percent also thought that these benefits would outweigh any risk to privacy and security.

Other studies have conducted focus groups, which allow for a more in-depth discussion of attitudes toward privacy. The focus group results more clearly point to attitudes that combine awareness of the potential benefits from HIE and the risk posed to privacy. Simon et al. (2009) conducted focus groups involving 64 participants in several rural towns participating in the Massachusetts eHealth Collaborative (MAeHC). Participants' privacy concerns focused on access by people who do not need the information for treatment or through security breaches, but the participants were not concerned about their providers having access to sensitive information. The discussions revealed broad endorsement of the potential benefits of HIE to improve health care. When asked to review and discuss the consent form currently being used by the collaborative, participants wanted well-designed information sent to them before they were asked to provide consent. The Agency for Healthcare Research and Quality commissioned a study to conduct 20 focus groups around the country in 2009 (Westat, 2009). The first half of these two-hour discussions was designed to educate participants about health IT issues, and the second half focused on the role of consumers in the design and use of health IT. As in the Massachusetts study, participants believed that health IT would improve health care, but a large majority expressed concerns about privacy and security. Believing that individuals own their PHI, nearly all partici-

---

[7]   Similarly, Patel et al. (2012) found that 83 percent of the patients of physicians participating in a Rochester, N.Y. RHIO supported use of HIE.

pants supported individual control over how data are shared and used, although they were not optimistic that they would get control. Many wanted the opportunity to consent in advance, even for sharing their information for emergencies.

People are clearly concerned about privacy, and they want to have control over who has access to their health information and for what purpose. Recent reports of the accidental release of electronic financial information and social networking data as well as high-profile security breaches of financial and health data may have increased people's awareness of these risks. Patients are willing to having their PHI shared, but they want it to be secure and to have a say in who has access.

Framework for Privacy and Security

Recognizing the importance of addressing privacy concerns in maintaining the patient and provider trust necessary for realizing the potential benefits of HIE, DHHS and others have developed frameworks that identify privacy protection and information security principles that HIOs should follow. The DHHS framework (Office of the National Coordinator for Health Information Technology, 2008), built on previous federal and international efforts, lays out eight principles or fair information practices to guide individuals and organizations in the health care sector participating in a network to exchange information.[8] The principles describe individuals' rights with respect to their PHI:

- access to the information through a simple and timely means in a readable format
- a means to dispute the accuracy or integrity of their information and correct it or have their dispute recorded
- transparency about policies, procedures, and technologies that affect them or their PHI

---

[8]   See also McGraw and Egerman (2010).

- reasonable opportunity to make informed choices about the collection, use, and disclosure of their information[9]
- collection, use, and disclosure of information only to the extent necessary for specified purposes and never to discriminate
- reasonable steps to ensure that information collected is complete, accurate, and up-to-date
- protection of the information with reasonable safeguards to ensure confidentiality, integrity, and accessibility and to prevent unauthorized access, use, or disclosure
- monitoring of the implementation of these principles and the reporting and mitigation of non-adherence and breaches, including notification of individuals put at substantial risk by privacy violations.

These principles for ensuring privacy protection for health information are consistent with the principles that guide federal requirements for privacy protection of other personal information. For example, the Fair Credit Reporting Act (15 U.S.C. § 1681 et seq.), enacted before HIPAA in 1970, gives consumers the rights to access their credit reports, dispute information in the reports, and limit disclosure for certain purposes (e.g., marketing). The act also prohibits the disclosure of health information for employment purposes. Similarly, the Privacy Act of 1974 (5 USC § 552a) regulates the collection, use, and disclosure of personal information by federal agencies. The Privacy Act restricts disclosure without the individual's consent and gives individuals the right to access their information, request amendment of incorrect information, and obtain a record of the disclosures of their information.

Similar privacy frameworks for health information have also been developed by two other groups: (1) a consortium of California organizations concerned about trust in and the privacy and security of electronic PHI, organized by Consumers Union and the Center for Democracy and Technology, and sponsored by the California Health-

---

[9] Although not stated explicitly in this framework, individual choice should include the option to revoke authorization or consent to collect, use, or disclose information. This topic is addressed in more detail in the discussion of meaningful patient consent in Chapter Three.

Care Foundation (2011); and (2) the Markle-sponsored Connecting for Health Public-Private Collaboration,[10] which involves more than 100 organizations drawn from the provider community, government, and industry with expertise in care delivery, technology, privacy, and the consumer experience. One notable principle included by the California consortium is local control—keeping PHI under the control of the patient or health care organization responsible for the individual's care. The Markle Collaboration included legal and financial remedies to address security breaches or privacy violations among the general policy principles in its framework.

The Markle Collaboration has developed a complementary set of technology principles, two of which address the subject of this report:

- "All health information exchange, including in support of the delivery of care and the conduct of research and public health reporting, must be conducted in an environment of trust, based upon conformance with appropriate requirements for patient privacy, security, confidentiality, integrity, audit, and *informed consent.*"
- "Accuracy in identifying both a patient and his or her records with little tolerance for error is an essential element of health information exchange. There must also be feedback mechanisms to help organizations to fix or "clear" their data in the event that errors are discovered."

Summary

We found widespread consensus on the principles that should guide HIE, including consent for HIE and accuracy in linking EHR information to patients. However, as we will discuss in the next chapter, there is less consensus about specific approaches to implementing these principles. Furthermore, despite public emphasis on the need for pri-

---

[10] Markle Foundation, undated.

vacy in HIE, many health care organizations that are sharing data externally have yet to implement basic privacy protections, such as employee privacy training, data sharing agreements with all participants, or the monitoring of business associates (Health Research Institute, 2011). Similarly, an evaluation of HIE policies and procedures at five California health care organizations concluded that none came close to complying with all the principles developed for that state (Miller, 2012). In the following chapters, we discuss privacy implications as well as other technical, organizational, and social issues of informed consent and patient identity management.

CHAPTER THREE

Patient Consent for Health Information Exchange

Policy and Legal Background

As noted in Chapter Two, electronic HIE heightens concerns about the privacy of patient health information. Recording and transmitting patient information electronically make it very easy to request and send patient health information, and exchange models involving transmission of PHI among third parties, such as HIOs, increase risks of disclosure and misuse (McGraw and Egerman, 2010). Patient consent or authorization for HIE is central to the issue of privacy, yet there is often ambiguity and controversy about the meaning of *consent* and mechanisms for obtaining it. For example, responses to requests for public comment on the proposed HIPAA rule revealed that many individuals felt that they "own" their health records and should be asked for permission to release PHI with every request; these sentiments are supported by privacy rights organizations but not by current law and practice ("Federal Register," 2000).

There are a number of laws and regulations regarding patient consent for disclosure of PHI at the federal and state level. In the next section, we summarize some of these requirements.

Federal Regulations

The HIPAA Privacy Rule (45 CFR Parts 160 and 164), issued by DHHS, addresses the disclosure and use of individuals' PHI that is or has been maintained or transmitted electronically by covered entities. Covered entities include health care providers, health plans, health care clearinghouses such as billing services, and business associates, i.e., individuals or organizations that perform activities involving the use of PHI or its disclosure to a covered entity. HITECH extended privacy regulations to business associates that regularly access or transmit PHI, such as RHIOs and HIOs. It also requires patient consent for disclosure of information about care when the patient is paying for the care (see Chapter Two for a summary of other requirements set forth in HITECH).[1]

The Privacy Rule attempts to create a balance between safeguarding individuals' privacy and allowing for the disclosure and use of information to promote health care quality and efficiency. There are several situations or activities for which covered entities can disclose PHI without first obtaining authorization from the patient.[2] Of particular relevance for this report is the disclosure of PHI without prior consent for the purposes of treatment, payment, or health care operations. Treatment includes providing, coordinating, or managing health care and related services by health care providers. The concept of health care operations is defined broadly. It includes, for example, a variety of evaluation activities, such as quality improvement efforts, credentialing/accreditation, medical reviews, and business planning. An important principle of the Privacy Rule is that of "minimum necessary" use

---

[1] HIPAA distinguishes between authorization and consent. Authorization is required for uses and disclosures of PHI that are not otherwise permitted or required under the Privacy Rule. Authorization must be written and contain a number of required elements, such as the a description of the information to be used and disclosed, the entity authorized to make the use or disclosure, the recipient, an expiration date, and, in some cases, the purposes for which the information may be used or disclosed. Consent refers to written permission to use or disclose PHI to carry out treatment, payment, and health care operations. Generally, covered entities are permitted but not required to obtain consent, and they are free to design the consent process as they see fit.

[2] Other activities for which patient authorization is not required include disclosure to the individual patient (unless authorization is required for access or to account for disclosures); opportunity to agree or object (e.g., informal patient consent may be obtained for notification purposes such as informing a family member about the patient's condition); incidental to an otherwise permitted use and disclosure (disclosure that occurs as a consequence of other permitted use and disclosure as long as the information being shared was the minimum necessary and the organization has adopted reasonable data safeguarding procedures per the Privacy Rule); public interest and benefit activities; and creation of a limited data set for the purposes of research, public health, or health care operations.

and disclosure, such that covered entities must make reasonable efforts to use, disclose, and request only the minimum amount of PHI needed to accomplish the intended purpose. Covered entities must also provide reasonable safeguards for individuals' PHI.

The Privacy Rule does require patient authorization for disclosure of an individual's psychotherapy notes, even within the same health care organization (with some exceptions, such as use by the covered entity to provide treatment or legal proceedings brought about by the patient against the covered entity), and for marketing communications for health-related products or services. These restrictions on disclosure of PHI do not apply in the case of military personnel when the disclosure is for activities "deemed necessary by appropriate military command authorities to assure the proper execution of the military mission."

The Clinical Laboratory Improvement Amendment (CLIA) generally restricts release of lab test results only to "authorized persons" and, if applicable, the person responsible for using the test results and the laboratory that requested the test. "Authorized person" is generally understood to be the person who ordered the test, however, the meaning of "person responsible for using the test results" is not clear, and state law influences who is authorized to receive this information. CLIA is more restrictive than HIPAA, which permits covered entities to disclose PHI to other providers for treatment without patient permission.

Federal regulations on the Confidentiality of Alcohol and Drug Abuse Patient Records (42 CFR Part 2) has confidentiality requirements that apply to alcohol and drug abuse treatment programs that receive federal assistance. These regulations require written patient consent for disclosure of information[3] and prohibit individuals or organizations that have received information from redisclosing it without patient permission. Consent is "opt-in," and consent forms have a

[3]   With some exceptions, including disclosure to medical personnel in the cases of bona fide emergencies; for some law enforcement purposes (although the information cannot be used to initiate or substantiate criminal charges against the patient); and for scientific research, evaluations, or audits if patient identities are concealed.

number of required elements, including program name, patient name, recipient name, how much and what kind of information will be disclosed, signature of the patient or authorized signatory (e.g., parent or guardian for a minor), and the date on which consent was signed. To be considered a program, a provider or unit/group within a general medical facility must specialize in substance abuse diagnosis, treatment, or referral. The VA has substance abuse programs under this definition, but the MTFs do not.

The Pensions, Bonuses, and Veterans' Relief regulations govern disclosure of the identity, diagnosis, prognosis, or treatment of any VHA patient with regard to drug abuse, alcohol abuse or alcoholism, infection with HIV/AIDs, and sickle cell anemia (38 CFR Part 1 §§1.460 through 1.499). Requests for medical records that include this information require written consent from the patient, with some exceptions, such as those that apply to Title 42 (see Bouhaddou et al., 2011), and additional exceptions pertaining to public health. Like Title 42, recipients of this information may not re-disclose it, and they may not use it for purposes other than that for which disclosure was made.

Title 42 and Title 38 exempt DoD and the VA from their prohibitions on the exchange of the covered health information for military personnel and veterans. However, HIE with civilian providers or for other beneficiaries is subject to the prohibitions in these two acts.

State Regulations

There are myriad state laws regarding the disclosure of PHI. Federal law, such as HIPAA and HITECH, preempt any conflicting state laws. However, state laws and regulations that impose stricter requirements on the handling of PHI still apply.

Dimitropoulos and Rizk (2009) reviewed state law on this topic. As they describe, there are numerous and varied state laws, and some regulations are unclear and subject to varying interpretations. In general, Dimitropoulos and Rizk note the following:

- Many states permit disclosure of general clinical information, HIV-related information, and genetics-related information without patient permission for treatment purposes, but some states

require permission for at least one of these three types of information (HIV information in particular), and a few states require
patient permission for all three types of information.

- Many states have adopted the requirements of 42 CFR Part 2
  regarding the disclosure of information related to substance
  abuse, and some states impose these requirements on non–
  federally assisted programs.
- Few states permit clinical laboratories to disclose test results to
  providers other than those who requested the tests.
- Regulations and statutes regarding mental health information
  were the most complex, detailed, and varied.

It is beyond the scope of this report to describe state law in detail.
The central issue with respect to patient consent is that electronic transmission facilitates the exchange of PHI and the potential for information to be exchanged across states, yet states have different disclosure
requirements. Pritts and Connor (2007) describe several solutions to
this problem:

- Adopt a federal standard (e.g., the HIPAA Privacy Rule) that
  would preempt state law.
- Adopt a national policy that allows individuals to have lim-
  ited, uniform control over the disclosure of certain types of
  information.
- Develop a uniform act for health information disclosure.
- Enter into interstate compacts.
- Develop standardized rules for disclosure that could be used in an
  automated HIE system (use of this approach for HIE within an
  HIO is described in more detail later in this report).

However, there are downsides to many of these approaches. For
example, a preemptive federal regulation would nullify state laws that
have stricter regulations regarding the disclosure of PHI for treatment
purposes. A policy that gives patients uniform control over disclosure
would limit HIE in states that allow providers to disclose PHI for treatment without patient permission. Given variation in state regulations,

Pritts and Connor are pessimistic about the feasibility of a uniform act. They conclude that any solution that regulates HIE across states would require more standardized rules that differ from current regulations reflecting local preferences in some states.

Consent Principles

Valid, informed consent consists of five elements: disclosure, capacity or competence, understanding or comprehension, voluntariness, and consent or decision (del Carmen and Joffe, 2005; Faden and Beauchamp, 1986). Disclosure means that the consenter has the information needed to make an autonomous decision. Capacity refers to the consenter's ability to understand the information and to make judgments about the potential consequences of his or her decision. Understanding reflects the consenter's comprehension of the information provided (e.g., consent or authorization form). Voluntariness reflects the consenter's right to make a decision freely, without external pressure or coercion. Consent or decision reflects the consenter's authorization, e.g., for HIE. Mechanisms for the decision include the consent or authorization form and discussions with the relevant "agent" or "gatekeeper," e.g., the health care provider. These principles support autonomy, which is a central premise of informed consent. For decisions to be autonomous, the health care provider must ensure that the consenter acts intentionally and voluntarily and understands the information provided.

Patient Consent Methods

Types of Patient Consent

A white paper prepared for the ONC delineates five models of consent for HIE (Goldstein and Rein, 2010a):

- *No consent:* HIE occurs automatically; there is no opportunity for the patient to consent to participate.[4] In the three VLER pilots described earlier (Tidewater, Spokane, and Puget Sound), the MTFs use a no-consent model for disclosing information for active duty and retired military patients to another VLER site (whereas to ensure that the consent requirements in Title 38 and Title 42 are met, the VA requires active consent for disclosing information for veterans). Typically, no-consent models would only be found in states with no additional provisions for HIE beyond federal HIPAA requirements. In some cases, an HIO may have a requirement that patients are notified regarding their participation and informed of the purposes of the information exchange, which is a principle of the privacy frameworks described in Chapter One of this report. Goldstein and Rein also describe an alternative in which there is no opportunity for patients to consent to which information flows into the system, but have some control regarding how the information can be used, such as who receives it and for what purposes.
- *Opt-out consent:* Eligibility of HIE for all or some types of data (e.g., labs) occurs by default. The patient must respond if he or she does not wish to participate. Survey data from 196 health exchange initiatives revealed that most use opt-out consent at the provider or organizational level (eHealth Initiative, 2011). Most of these HIOs are in states with no requirements for consent beyond HIPAA. DoD uses opt-out consent in that patients may request restrictions on uses and disclosures of their medical record, but the MTF is not required to agree to the restrictions if they are difficult to accommodate or if they conflict with other policies of Army Regulation 40-66.

---

[4] Consistent with HIPAA, the TRICARE Privacy Notice describes an option for patients to request restrictions on disclosure of their PHI for treatment, payment, or health care operations. The request must be made in writing and need not be approved if not considered in the interest of the patient or the MHS or if it cannot be reasonably implemented. This procedure has not been automated at this time, and none of the VLER pilot sites reported having patients who had successfully exercised this option.

- *Opt-out consent with exceptions:* This model allows for some level of granularity or data segmentation. In this model, all or some types of data exchange occur by default, but the patient has the authority to set limits in terms of the types of data, the specific providers or organizations to receive the data, and/or specific purposes of data use. The eHealth Initiative survey results indicate that many health exchange initiatives enable patients to opt out by data type, encounter, sending organization, data field (e.g., demographic information), or data sensitivity. However, the survey did not reveal how organizations implement these patient preferences.
- *Opt-in consent:* The default is no data exchange; written authorization is required for participation. In most cases, opt-in consent involves all-or-nothing data exchange; the patient cannot restrict certain types of information from being exchanged. The decision not to participate can be overridden in some cases, such as for emergency care.
- *Opt-in consent with restrictions:* This model is similar to an opt-in model, but patients can impose limits on data exchange based on types of data, recipients, purposes of data use, and access (e.g., viewing or disclosing the data). Again, the eHealth Initiative survey documents the use of opt-in consent based on particular categories (see opt-out consent with exceptions above), but the means of implementation are not described.

Studies comparing opt-in and opt-out consent for health care purposes find much higher participation rates using opt-out procedures (Junghans et al., 2005; Stanley, Fraser, and Cox, 2003). For example, Junghans et al. conducted a double-blind randomized control trial of the type of consent for recruitment in research among 510 angina patients in two general practices in England. The study showed significantly higher rates of recruitment (defined by clinic attendance) in the opt-out arm (50 percent) than in the opt-in arm (38 percent). There were also differences in the characteristics of respondents in that those who opted in were generally healthier than those in the opt-out group.[5]

Trade-offs Among Consent Approaches

There are trade-offs among the types of consent described above. Opt-out consent, as it is often implemented in organizations, can yield high rates of participation because the onus is on the patient to respond. In addition, even if the provider is diligent in contacting patients, the meaning of a nonresponse can be ambiguous, leading to questions about disclosure (did the patient receive the information?), capacity (did the patient have the ability to understand the information?), and understanding (did the patient comprehend the information?). In contrast, opt-in consent can be more labor-intensive for the provider (and, in some cases, for the patient, if he or she needs to respond by mail, for example), and participation rates may be lower because explicit authorization is required of each patient and because some patients may refuse to participate. Opt-in consent methods appear to offer greater privacy protections for patients at a cost of potentially lower rates of participation in an HIO and therefore reduced opportunities for improvement in quality and efficiency of care afforded by HIE (Tripathi et al., 2009). In fact, some states, organizations, or other entities endorse or permit only opt-in consent (Heinze et al., 2011, Tripathi et al., 2009). Thus, there are ethical arguments about opt-in and opt-out approaches; some people endorse opt-out consent because higher participation rates mean potentially better individual and public health outcomes; others argue that opt-out approaches violate basic principles of informed consent.

Implementation of Consent Models

ONC's HIT policy committee formed a "Tiger Team" to study issues of privacy and security in HIE (McGraw and Egerman, 2010). The Tiger Team asserted that both opt-in and opt-out approaches can be

---

[5] A pilot study using opt-in consent (Bouhaddou et al., 2011), described later in this report, also found differences in patient characteristics in that patients who opted in were older than those who did not respond. The authors concluded that older patients might have more health problems and therefore might benefit more from HIE than would younger patients.

implemented poorly; for example, by implementing opt-in consent with limited education or by using opt-out consent with limited notice or time for the patient to make a decision to participate. While we agree that both opt-in and opt-out consent can be implemented poorly, we argue that an opt-out procedure, even if carefully designed, can never be as effective as a careful opt-in procedure. Because many patients do not come into the office on a regular basis, it is difficult to ensure disclosure, capacity, and understanding for all patients using an opt-out approach. As a result, opt-out approaches may not reflect voluntary decisionmaking on the part of patients. One major teaching hospital recently decided to implement an opt-in consent procedure for these reasons (Halamka, 2012).

The Tiger Team recommended "meaningful, revocable" consent for HIE other than direct provider-to-provider exchange. These recommendations apply to Stage 1 meaningful use and have been incorporated into Medicare's Care Organization final rule ("Federal Register," 2011). That is, assuming that fair information practices are followed, data exchange for treatment does not require consent beyond the requirements of current laws or "customary practice" (McGraw and Egerman, 2010). However, when the decision to exchange PHI is not within the control of the provider or the provider's health care arrangement (e.g., as in the case of an HIO that operates a centralized model), patients should be able to give meaningful consent subject to the following conditions:

- advance notice and sufficient time to make a decision to participate, aside from when urgent care is needed
- it is not compelled, e.g., is not a condition for receiving services
- full transparency and education, including a clear explanation of the choices and consequences
- it is commensurate with the sensitivity of the activity, e.g., more specific mechanisms for more sensitive activities
- it is consistent with reasonable patient expectations for privacy, health, and safety
- it is revocable at any time.

The Tiger Team concluded also that the individual who directly treats the patient, typically the provider, holds the "trust relationship" (p. 12) and should be responsible for educating the patient about how their PHI is collected, used, and shared. This is consistent with survey data indicating that most patients want to make decisions about sharing their health information with their physicians, and often also with family members (Dimitropoulos et al., 2011).

A recent trend in approaches to obtaining patient consent involves a shift in control of the process from providers to patients. One impetus for this change lies in federal regulations requiring consent to obtain specific types of information, such as that relating to substance abuse and, in the case of veterans, other types of health information. The Healthcare Information Technology Standards Panel (HITSP) describes standards for a consent creator system that enables patients to specify and manage consent directives determining how their PHI can be collected and used within, for example, an HIO (HITSP, 2009a). A consent directive is a record of the consumer's privacy policy that grants or withholds consent for PHI based on the recipient; the type of data operations (e.g., collect, access); the instance and type of PHI; the purpose, such as treatment, payment, or research; the particular conditions (e.g., if the patient is unconscious) and contexts (e.g., emergencies); and over what period (HITSP, 2009a). These standards are based on security and privacy principles derived from major federal and state laws and regulations (HITSP, 2009b).

The VA is establishing a capability through its personal health record (My HealtheVet) to allow users to specify preferences that partially automate the authorization process for sharing health information with NwHIN partners.[6] Others also describe patient or person-centric electronic consent management systems for an HIO (Heinze et al., 2011; Mork, Rosenthal, and Stanford, 2011). For example, the prototype described by Mork, Rosenthal, and Stanford provides a single location that allows patients to specify their preferences for HIE nationwide and covers a variety of uses of PHI, such as emergency care and research. Each patient has a unique ID in the consent service that

---

[6] U.S. Department of Veteran's Affairs, 2012.

he or she is required to provide to each provider. Patients can specify their preferences once (and can revise their preferences); preferences are then applied to each request for PHI. Mork, Rosenthal, and Stanford describe how the service can be used in both an automated and manual fashion with providers' electronic or paper records.

Person-centric approaches offer numerous benefits to consumers and providers. Centralized consent offers consumers control over who gets their PHI, for what purposes, and over what time frame. It also provides one location where consumers can track their consent preferences, which may otherwise be difficult or impossible to do if they sign separate agreements on a provider-by-provider basis, particularly when practices change hands or when providers leave practices. A centralized service is also advantageous to providers by eliminating the need to maintain records of patients' consent preferences or to track down patients to obtain permission to use or disclose data in unanticipated situations (Mork, Rosenthal, and Stanford, 2011).

Despite these advantages, consumer-centric approaches also have many challenges to overcome. For example, the system described by Mork, Rosenthal, and Stanford requires providers to have the means to store and access the consent service ID in their systems. Moreover, successful adoption depends on a variety of sociotechnical factors. Notably, this system shifts primary responsibility for identity management from providers to patients. While this may be a benefit for patients who want to control how their PHI is used, some patients may not want this responsibility or be capable of managing it. More important, if patients put restrictions on the content of the health information that can be exchanged, then the provider's system must be capable of granular HIE or the provider must be willing to filter the patients' data manually. As Mork, Rosenthal, and Stanford note, providers may be inclined to refuse to process requests for patient health information with privacy constraints (which arguably is a primary reason for a person-centric approach). Provider resistance and other challenges to meeting patient preferences for HIE are discussed in the section entitled "Granular Consent" below.

Experiences with Consent for Health Information Exchange

Field studies documenting organizations' experiences obtaining consent for HIE point to the need for aggressive patient outreach and consumer-friendly authorization procedures. For example, Greenhalgh et al. (2010) describe implementation of a summary care record (SCR) for 29.8 million patients in the National Programme for Health Information Technology in England. Consent for participation used an opt-out approach. Letters were sent to patients describing the SCR and explaining how to opt out; fewer than 1 percent responded. Low opt-out rates were attributed to several reasons, including a purported lack of balance in the information provided, letters that were discarded without being read or that were not understood by patients, and a confusing opt-out process. In fact, in earlier pilots of the SCR, most patients were not aware of the SCR and did not recall receiving information about it, despite an aggressive marketing campaign for the program (Greenhalgh et al., 2008). Subsequently, the consent process was changed to an opt-in model presented by clinicians at the point of care. Even after the change, however, there were concerns that patients were not given sufficient time to consider their options regarding participation.

As we described above, the VA established an opt-in consent procedure for the VLER pilot, but DoD has not implemented consent. In our interviews, we asked about plans for consent for HIE by DoD when VLER moves beyond the pilot phase. Interviewees consistently acknowledged the importance of addressing consent for HIE, especially for dependents, but there is little in the way of consent plans or policy at this stage in VLER development. Consistent with the VA's policy on consent, the VLER site in San Diego piloted a patient consent process to invite veterans to opt-in to electronic HIE (Bouhaddou et al., 2011).[7] Shared patients (n = 1,144) of the VA and Kaiser Permanente were sent personalized letters explaining the benefits of electronic HIE along with VA and Kaiser authorization forms, instruc-

---

[7] Results of identifying and matching patients are described in Chapter Four of this report.

tions, and a self-addressed stamped envelope. Patients were informed that they were free to opt in, that they could revoke authorization at any time, and that the VA and Kaiser were the only organizations that would exchange data. Patients received an automatic phone reminder one week after the invitations were mailed.

A total of 501 patients responded, for a participation rate of 44 percent, which Bouhaddou et al. describe as "very large" (2011, p. 140). However, 25 percent of the respondents had invalid authorizations due to mismatches between protected conditions the respondents agreed to exchange in the authorization forms and those that were present in the patient's records, as well as due to missing signatures or other information.[8] In addition, all VA authorization forms had to be verified manually against the patients' charts, a process that does not scale.

In contrast, the MAeHC conducted pilot projects to implement EHRs in three communities and link them to allow providers to exchange patient health information (Tripathi et al., 2009). The pilots involved 597 primary care providers and over 500,000 patients. Patient consent was seen as the central privacy issue and was a focus of consumer councils that had a critical role in governance for the collaborative. The pilots used opt-in consent and obtained a 90 percent participation rate.[9]

There are a number of factors that may account for the success of the MAeHC pilots and that are important lessons for other HIE efforts:

---

[8]   To be valid, each of 38 protected conditions that were checked off in the VA authorization form had to be present in the patient's medical record; likewise, protected conditions in the record had to be marked on the authorization form. Subsequently, a revised VA form was approved for NwHIN in which the patient authorizes disclosure of conditions whether or not they are present in the record.

[9]   Three factors drove the decision to use opt-in consent. First, stakeholders adopted a conservative approach due to uncertainty about privacy laws, as Massachusetts has strict regulations mandated by case law rather than by a specific statute. Second, opt-out consent was not feasible because the system architecture used a centralized data repository rather than a decentralized approach. Third, consumers were concerned that an opt-out approach could result in inadvertent disclosure of patients' health information.

- a focus on privacy and consent as a major design criterion rather than as an afterthought
- a governance process involving patients and users
- negotiation of decisions about what health information to share in order to strike a balance between providing clinically useful data and preventing large numbers of patients from refusing to opt in
- implementation of a carefully designed marketing and communications plan to recruit patients.

More specifically, MAeHC hired a health literacy specialist and marketing firm to assist in patient recruitment. Focus groups evaluated recruitment materials, including consent forms, educational brochures, and frequently asked questions. Common suggestions made in the focus groups that influenced the marketing approach included

- relate HIE to the issues that consumers are most frustrated with, i.e., inconvenience and the high cost of health care
- rely on the clinician to be the primary means of communication about HIE
- address the points most important to consumers up front, which included convenience, safety, ease of management of health information, and patient control through opt-in (rather than, for example, quality of care)
- clearly describe the risks and mitigating strategies, e.g., for security concerns
- use "professional" marketing materials that are memorable to patients (rather than "serious" materials that have a noncommercial appearance).

Granular Consent

The "opt-in with restrictions" and "opt-out with exceptions" models of consent are also known as granular consent. Granular consent enables patients to express their preferences regarding sharing their health information, which, in their report for ONC, Goldstein and Rein (2010b) argue is central to supporting personal autonomy and engaging consumers in HIE efforts. Implementing granular consent requires data segmentation, or methods that limit data capture, access, and/or use based on factors such as recipient, purpose, duration, and the content of patient health information. However, there are numerous challenges to data segmentation to support granular consent. We review several of these challenges here; for a more comprehensive analysis, see the Goldstein and Rein report.

The national provider IDs mandated by HIPAA can be used to control patient information based on recipient, as long as all of the records have this ID. Whereas this sort of restriction sounds straightforward to implement in principle, there are many potential technical barriers, such as constraints imposed by legacy systems, as well as "people" barriers, e.g., does the patient need to know their providers' IDs, are they presented with a drop-down menu of providers in their area, or does the system include a lookup (which requires provider identity matching)?

Patients may wish to restrict access to their health information based on the purpose of data use. Under HIPAA, patient authorization is not required for the purposes of treatment, payment, or health care operations, but patients may request limits on disclosure, and state laws may be more restrictive. In addition, patient permission may be required for other purposes, such as marketing, research, and public health reporting. Restrictions based on purpose (e.g., treatment, marketing, research) might be implemented by pre-coding so that the provider can indicate the purpose(s) and these can be matched against the purposes for which the patient has given consent. However, pre-coding by itself does not ensure that the codes are interpreted properly and the information is shared only as the patient intended.

Duration can refer either to the length of time to which authorization applies (after which point the patient must re-consent or consent lapses) or to the dates during which data may or may not be shared. Clearly, after consent lapses or is revoked, information about care cannot be shared. Many consent forms also specify the period to which the consent applies (e.g., for data about the patient obtained prior to the consent date). Less clear is what data the provider has access to after a patient revokes consent, e.g., can a provider retrieve information for care that was provided prior to the date of consent withdrawal?

Different consent models, as well as federal and state law, have led ONC to pursue the development of content-based granular consent, which requires data segmentation capabilities that allow only some content to be disclosed. However, the current state of EHRs does not support effective data segmentation based on content. Thus, patients typically need to give blanket opt-in or opt-out consent to disclose content.

Some EHRs enable providers to suppress transmission of specific codes in the medical record or to set access controls by the episode, encounter, or location of care (McGraw and Egerman, 2010). However, segmentation methods that rely on provider behavior, such as tagging sensitive content or entering information into particular fields, are likely to fail. Clinical documents used for HIE also have standards for fields that can be used for granular consent, but the availability of such technology does not ensure that it is actually used. For example, mental health fields in the continuity of care document (CCD) standard used for HIE include flags for sections of the document that allow role-based access to section content (Ferranti et al., 2006; Hsieh, 2011). However there is no way to ensure that sensitive information is limited to those fields. By some estimates, as much as 50 percent of the clinical information in EHRs is captured in the unstructured text of the clinical narrative, even when a system is provided for structuring content that might be used for standardization and segmentation (Miller, 2012; Turchin et al., 2009; Skentzos et al., 2011). In fact, rather than adhering to the detailed structures supported by HIE and CCD standards, HIE commonly consists of unstructured information and notes that are difficult to parse meaningfully for purposes of privacy or communication (Unertl et al., 2011). Indeed, the inability to reliably guarantee compliance with Title 38 due to potential inclusion of PHI has led to difficulties in consent management for demonstration projects intended to facilitate information exchange between the VA and private providers (Bouhaddou et al., 2011). Likewise, the use of unstructured clinical notes poses a problem for the automated detection of HIPAA-restricted identifiers.

Many EHRs have the capability to suppress psychotherapy notes (narrative). However, it is difficult to ensure that all information generated from a particular episode or about mental health treatment (such as prescription information) is suppressed. In addition, given the ways that many providers use fields in their EHRs, restricting the transmission of narrative text may also prevent the exchange of other health information needed for clinical care. Research is needed to design systems that encourage meaningful text structuring to support patient consent preferences (Mandl et al., 2001).

Research on automated text processing uses natural language processing (NLP) and machine learning methods for structuring and filtering data, similar to the procedures used for redaction in classified documents. While these approaches have the advantage of not requiring workflow redesign for providers, current approaches are not capable of redacting information that is not codified in standard ways, and methods are still evolving (McGraw and Egerman, 2010). In addition, algorithms for automated processing are subject to false positives and false negatives, with obvious trade-offs between these types of errors.

The research intended to impose structure using NLP (for example, Hazlehurst et al., 2005) includes few empirical studies that have examined technical approaches to clinical data segmentation specifically for privacy purposes. Researchers have found that the most conservative filters could reliably redact HIV information with limited redaction of other health information (Staddon, Golle, and Zimny, 2007; Chow, Golle, and Straddon, 2008). These algorithms might be applied in a fully automated process upon the transfer of unstructured text data, as alerts for patient management systems, or even before a document is closed, to remind a provider that he or she may need to apply structured privacy flags to part of the note. All of these scenarios present needs for both computer science and usability research.

Summary

We anticipate that a number of changes in mechanisms for consent will be needed to support the VLER. DoD will need the capacity to record and implement patients' restrictions on disclosure of PHI when they are approved under the current opt-out procedure. However, current methods for implementing granular consent are in their infancy.

In addition, we expect that it may be difficult to proceed with VLER without a meaningful consent procedure that reflects the principles proposed by the Tiger Team. Although HIPAA allows providers to share patient health information for the purposes of treatment, payment, and operations without patient authorization, we expect that many civilian providers may not be able or willing to do so, particularly those providers who reside in states with additional requirements for consent beyond the federal requirements. DoD may conclude that the best approach is to follow in the VA's footsteps and develop an online patient consent management system for non–active duty beneficiaries. DoD also faces some unique challenges with respect to consent for HIE, such as consent for the exchange of pre-accession PHI for an active duty member who was a dependent prior to joining the military.

Proactive research, carried out in the unique context of the military, would inform the development of future consent policy and practice as well as the design of next-generation health IT systems that will need to handle consent restrictions, if only for care provided by non-DoD providers. In the concluding chapter, we present specific needs for research to support these goals.

CHAPTER FOUR

Patient Identity Management

PHI is linked to individual patients through a number of identifiers, such as name, address, email address, phone number, a unique patient identifying number (e.g., Social Security number [SSN] or a number maintained for use only in health care), health plan or other account number, birthdate, and personal characteristics such as gender. Identifiers link information to the individual patient when the information is stored or retrieved by a single provider with a health IT system and/or exchanged across systems by providers treating the same patient. Non-unique, out-of-date, or incorrect identifiers can cause two types of errors:

- false negatives: failure to find a patient's information when it in fact exists
- false positives: finding information that is not, in fact, for the patient.[1]

False negatives decrease the benefits of EHRs because providers do not receive information that might improve the quality and cost-effectiveness of the care they deliver. False negatives lead to the creation of multiple identities and a split EHR, with some records linked to one identity and the other records linked to a second identity—for example, one with the name John Doe and another with the name John F.

---

[1] A true negative is correctly determining that the patient does not have any health information in the system. A true positive occurs when all the information for a patient, and only that information, is identified.

Doe. False positives can be dangerous if not caught and if they affect provider treatment decisions. Either type of error can reduce trust in the system from providers and patients.

Unique patient identifiers facilitate identity management, and many HIOs rely on preexisting identifiers known to be unique, such as SSN or email address. However, preexisting identifiers also identify individuals in financial, employer, government, and other IT systems, and the use of SSNs in particular in health IT systems could allow individuals' PHI to be linked to their other sensitive information (Greenberg and Ridgely, 2008). As directed by HIPAA, DHHS has established a framework for national unique identifiers for health care providers and health plans, but not yet for patients. Health care organizations assign unique identifiers to their patients, but the same person usually will not have the same identifier(s) across health care organizations. Where the same unique patient identifier is not used to link information to patients across health IT systems, a combination of other information (e.g., name, birthdate, address, gender) must be used for patient matching to exchange PHI across systems. These identifiers are more likely to be non-unique or entered with error and can become out of date.

Another key element of patient identity management is identity matching—i.e., identifying the same individual across health care organizations using the identifiers specified. Numerous methods are available, from simple deterministic algorithms that require an exact match on the specified identifiers to highly sophisticated probabilistic, hierarchical algorithms for which a threshold must be set to establish a match.

Together, the choice of identifiers and a matching algorithm constitute a patient matching approach and result in some rate of false negatives (including split EHRs) and false positives. Often, deciding what approach to use means trading off between the two types of errors. Approaches that have a very low probability of matching to the wrong person also often lead to false negatives—not successfully matching to information available from other providers. Maximizing the successful match rate often comes at a cost of increasing the false positive rate—linking to the wrong patient information. Unique and accurate patient identifiers as well as more effective matching algorithms can lower both types of errors.

In this section, we summarize the relevant federal and DoD policy, review different approaches to identifying and matching patients, and describe the experience of using these approaches in HIOs and VLER in particular. Published research on patient identity matching is limited; we summarize the results of studies that provide information relevant to the likely performance of approaches employing different identifiers and matching algorithms. However, we found no studies that have evaluated accuracy in an operating HIO.

Policy and Legal Background

HIPAA addressed patient identifiers indirectly by defining what makes health information not identifiable and therefore not subject to the provisions of the law. It specified a list of identifiers that must be removed to constitute a "safe harbor" method for de-identifying health information.[2] However, HIPAA does not address unstructured data that may identify the individual or that may be used with other information to infer identity. As the content of health information that can be exchanged expands, it may include identifying information imbedded in unstructured data, such as clinical notes.

HIPAA also included a provision directing DHHS to set up standards for a national health identifier for each individual, employer, health plan, and health care provider. In 2005, DHHS issued a rule for a unique provider identifier, which HIPAA requires providers to use for electronic claims billing, and a provider identifier registry system was subsequently implemented.[3] Proposed rules were recently published for the health plan identifier and also an identifier for other entities that are not individuals, health plans, or providers but need to be uniquely

---

[2] The list is designed to eliminate the possibility of combining information to infer an individual's identity. For example, it includes geographic subdivisions smaller than a state, except for the initial three digits of a zip code.

[3] MHS providers are required to obtain a national provider identity code.

identified in transactions. However, since 1999, Congress has with-held authority to expend funds on setting a standard for an individual identifier.

Until recently, DoD identified individuals by their SSNs. Fol-lowing up on an Office of Management and Budget directive to all federal agencies and citing the growing threat of identity theft, a policy directive to decrease the unnecessary use of SSNs was issued in March 2008 (Under Secretary of Defense [Personnel and Readiness], 2008). The policy defined acceptable uses of SSNs to include "those that are provided for by law, require interoperability with organizations beyond the DoD, or are required by operational necessities." It indicated that all uses of SSNs would be closely scrutinized and directed that use be expanded where possible of the DoD-created Electronic Data Inter-change Personal Identifier (EDI-PI), which was established in the 1990s for use with DoD's Common Access Card.[4] EDI-PI is the pri-mary identifier for all military personnel and other DoD beneficiaries in the Person Data Repository (PDR) maintained by DMDC.[5] The PDR also records SSN, name, and other personal information (e.g., birth date, gender, eligibility date), and the DoD Benefits Number (DBN)—another individual identifier that is used to access health care and other benefits. New DoD ID cards have the EDI-PI printed on the face and stored on the card electronically, and, for those eligible for benefits, the cards also have the DBN.

DMDC has been working with the VA to correlate its service member and veteran registries, and the VA has agreed to use the EDI-PI as the common declarative identifier in VLER, although it plans to retain its existing individual identifier for internal use. New service members and dependents are assigned an EDI-PI when they enter the military or become eligible for benefits, and older veterans without an EDI-PI are assigned one. The DoD and VA beneficiary records both

---

[4] The Common Access Card is an identification card for military personnel, civilian employees, and certain contract personnel that is used to authenticate access to DoD com-puters and facilities.

[5] The Person Data Repository is the renamed data file for the Defense Enrollment Eligibil-ity Reporting System (DEERS).

include the EDI-PI when it is assigned. There are 11 million individuals whose identities have been correlated (matched) so far,[6] and the two departments are developing a joint identity management architecture for the future.

To allow for patient matching with the VA and civilian providers, the MHS has requested and received an exemption to DoD policy on replacing SSNs, allowing for continued use of SSNs in health IT systems. Once EDI-PI is fully implemented in the VA, it will replace the SSN as the primary identifier used for patient identity matching between the two departments. However, SSNs will continue to be needed for HIE with civilian providers.[7]

Patient Identity Matching Methods

Choice of Identifiers

Without a national patient health identifier, HIOs must rely on identifiers that are recorded in the IT systems of their participating health care organizations. NwHIN has been designed to use any list of identifiers provided for matching to patient information from other participants.

The only universal identifier currently available for patients is the SSN, which is not recorded by all health care organizations in their patient directories or EHRs. Even if SSNs are used, they are not foolproof for patient matching. They may be mistyped into patient health records, the patient may not have their number when they arrive for care, or they may provide the wrong number. For example, parents sometimes provide their own information instead of their child's infor-

---

[6] DoD has 9.6 million service members and other beneficiaries currently eligible for benefits and a total of 44 million individuals in its repository, including members and dependents no longer eligible and civilian and contract personnel. The VA has over 15 million veterans registered. How many individuals will eventually be correlated for VLER is unclear, but it will be well over 11 million and will grow over time as new people become eligible.

[7] In the future, civilian providers will use DBNs instead of SSNs for TRICARE billing. EDI-PIs are added to the electronic claims records when the claims are adjudicated. DoD has not yet determined whether or on what basis it will disclose EDI-PIs to civilian providers. DoD is updating its health IT systems to support four-digit SSN search so that civilian providers do not have to use the full SSN.

mation when enrolling the child with a provider or providing information for a visit. Babies are not assigned SSNs or other identifying numbers at birth. And, as we discussed in Chapter Two, the use of SSNs increases privacy concerns because they are linked to other sensitive information, including financial information, and are known by employers. For this reason, some HIOs limit their use of SSNs in matching to the last four digits, and many patient-matching algorithms do not return the full SSN in reporting the results of a search for verification. However, research has shown that the first five digits can be identified using public records for 7 percent of individuals born between 1973 and 1988 and 44 percent of individuals born after 1988 (Acquisti and Gross, 2009). Using a method that identifies the two most likely sets of digits, the correct, complete SSN is revealed in one of these sets in 60 percent of cases. These are nationwide estimates; the percentages are much higher in small states. Thus, restricting use to the last four digits of the SSN still poses significant privacy concerns.

There are few other unique identifiers that are broadly available. Driver's license numbers are unique when combined with the state, but not everyone has a license. Also, driver's license numbers are not routinely recorded by providers, and they change with an interstate move—which is a particularly common occurrence among military beneficiaries. Medical plan numbers can be combined with the health plan identifier to create a unique identifier (using the national medical plan identifier when it is fully implemented), but this is also not available for all patients, and it probably changes more often than the driver's license number does. Like SSNs, even if unique, these identifiers are not foolproof.

Other identifiers—e.g., first name, last name, date of birth, gender, and address—are, at best, unique in combination. However, last names and addresses are subject to change, and providers face challenges in keeping the information up-to-date, especially if the patient has not sought care from them for a while.

Errors can be introduced for many other reasons (misspelling, typographical error, and inaccurate transcription due to poor handwriting or voice recording are common). It is not uncommon to find the same patient inconsistently identified even in a single provider's records, and consistency is harder to achieve across providers or health care organizations.

Duplicate Patient Identities

Inconsistencies in recording patient information within a health IT system lead to duplicate records. When there are duplicate records, patient matching between systems may reveal only the portion of information linked to one identity. An IBM analysis of 300 master patient index files at more than 112 hospitals across the United States revealed a mean 8 percent duplication rate. That is, on average, 8 percent of the individuals in these files had duplicated, or split, records (IBM, 2010). Thirty-three hospitals had duplication rates below 5 percent, but the eight hospitals with the highest rates (above 15 percent) had an average rate of 23 percent. According to IBM, its clients have suggested that the duplication rate should not exceed 2 percent, but this rate was achieved at only two hospitals. Regression analysis estimated the rate to be 4 percent for a file with 100,000 patients and 10 percent for a file with 3 million patients. This report also refers to an earlier study of over 150,000 patient-record pairs with a high likelihood of being for the same person but with differing identifying information. Two-thirds of the pairs were for women, and half of these had different last names. Three-fifths of all the pairs were missing the SSN in at least one record, and half of the rest had different SSNs. The IBM report concluded by noting that duplicate patient records pose risks to patient care, the value of investments in applications relying on linking patient data across time and across facilities or providers, patient and provider trust, regulatory compliance, and legal liability.

Hillestad et al. (2008) analyzed the Social Security Master Death File to estimate the probability of linking to the wrong individual *absent data errors or inconsistencies*. The probability of an incorrect match was one in 3,500 when first and last name, birth year, and zip code were used, but near zero when the last four digits of the SSN were added. Grannis, Overhage, and McDonald (2002) explored the ability to link patients in hospital registries to the death file. They found that one-third of the patient registry records lacked SSNs. Among the registry records with SSNs, the authors measured error rates of 9.2 percent in one hospital's registry and 4.7 percent in the other hospital's registry. The second hospital's rate was measured three years after a major effort to clean its registry data. Most SSN errors were caused by substitution of the SSN for another patient with the same last name (likely the primary insured family member) and typographical errors. About 40 percent of individuals with incorrect SSNs in the hospital registries could be matched using name and birth date. The researchers concluded that the best combination of identifiers was SSN, phonetically compressed first name, birth month, and gender; using these identifiers and a deterministic matching algorithm, they were able to correctly identify almost 90 percent of the matches with no false positives in this relatively small data set.

To investigate patient matching in EHRs, Durham et al. (2010) selected a clean subset of medical records from Vanderbilt University Medical Center and corrupted the data based on prior research measuring data entry error rates arising from optical character recognition, phonetic differences, and typographic mistakes. They found that only 14 percent of the records in their sample matched on all four identifiers used in the patient file after incorporating data entry errors.

To maintain the high-quality patient identity data needed for identity matching, health care organizations need to establish adequate processes for monitoring data quality and correcting errors (Dimitropoulos et al., 2009; Hillestad et al., 2008). Monitoring the rate at which new errors are introduced is valuable for identifying and correcting common sources of errors in an organization. To the extent that the rate of introduction of new errors can be decreased, ongoing data cleaning will require less effort.

Choice of Matching Algorithm

Matching algorithms generally fall into two categories: deterministic and probabilistic (Dimitropoulos et al., 2009). Deterministic models apply rules that stipulate which identifiers must agree to identify a patient match. They typically rely on an identifier, such as SSN, that is thought to be unique and confirm the match using other information (e.g., name, date of birth, gender). The rule may be a simple one requiring that all or some of the identifiers match. Alternatively, deterministic algorithms may be more advanced, for example, by employing more advanced matching logic or weighting schemes to give some identifying information priority over others in matching.

Probabilistic algorithms implement statistical or mathematical methods to identify matches, and there are a number of different methods that can be used. Typically, these matching algorithms are based on parameters that capture the characteristics of the identifying data to be used, including the inherent nature of the identifiers (e.g., likelihood of a change, difficulty in transcribing) and estimates of their data quality. Probabilistic algorithms determine whether a pair of records is for the same person based on the statistical chances of a match. Dimitropoulos et al. compare three statistical approaches and favor one of them—the Fellegi-Sunter algorithm—because it relies on an automated method for estimating parameters, is accurate, and produces measures of matching success. Internet search and data mining have led to active research developing and evaluating methods for use in the public and private sector, and the available technology for patient matching is likely to continue to advance.

Table 4.1 provides information about the patient matching approaches in use in 2009 by seven HIOs (Dimitropoulos et al., 2009). The table reports the number of HIOs using various types of identifiers, identity matching software types, and matching algorithms, and the full-time equivalent (FTE) hours each devotes to the manual review of patient matches. Although the HIOs varied in their stage of development and size of covered patient population (from 225,000 to 9.4 million unique persons), all had established patient matching procedures.

In the seven HIOs, identifiers typically included first and last name, date of birth, and gender, with SSN and address often added; use of other numerical identifiers was less common. Organizations using SSN matched on all digits but did not display the full SSN in reporting the results of a patient search. Duplicate patient identities were handled by adjusting the matching algorithm to eliminate duplicates where possible and through manual review. Most of the HIOs had an established process for correcting identifying information and updating clinical documents based on feedback from end users. The type of matching algorithm varied, but most used commercial software with

Table 4.1
Patient Matching Methods of Seven Health Information Organizations, 2009

	Matching Method	Number of HIOs
Identifier	Date of birth	7
	Zip code	7
	First name	7
	Last name	7
	Gender	6
	SSN	5
	Address	5
	Phone number	4
	Medical record number	3
	Insurance ID	2
	Middle name	2
	Driver's license number	1
	County	1
Matching software type	Commercial	5[a]
	Homegrown	2
Algorithm type	Probabilistic	4
	Deterministic	1
	Both	1
	Fuzzy match	1
Manual review staff	0.5–1.0 FTEs	3
	0 FTEs	2
	TBD	2

SOURCE: Dimitropoulos et al. (2009).

[a] Three HIOs have modified the commercial software.

some customization. It is unlikely that any of the HIOs used one of the highly sophisticated algorithms classified in an HIMSS white paper (2009) as "advanced." Although sophisticated algorithms outperform simpler algorithms in minimizing false negatives and false positives, even in the presence of data errors, they require considerable expertise and cost to set up and maintain.

Any patient matching method—deterministic or probabilistic/mathematical—can be implemented using different criteria for determining a patient identity match. For example, a simple deterministic algorithm can require that all identifiers exactly match or accept certain types of partial match. The criteria adopted will determine false negative and false positive rates. Given the identifiers and algorithm used, adopting criteria that increase the match rate (decrease the false negative rate) will also increase the false positive rate. Fearing the consequences of attaching one patient's health information to a different patient, many HIOs also establish criteria for identifying possible matches that can be further evaluated manually, referred to as disambiguation. Table 4.1 indicates that all but one of the seven HIOs in the Dimitropoulos et al. study assigned staff to manual review patient matches. Physicians may also check that the information they receive through HIE is for the right patient or have their clinic staff do so.

To scale to large databases and/or many HIE participants, the identity-matching algorithm must be efficient. A number of factors affect speed. More sophisticated algorithms using more information tend to take somewhat longer. Peer-to-peer matching in a federated system compares the patient information provided by the requesting provider with the information in records stored in the other participating provider's system. Peer-to-peer matching allows each provider organization to retain control of its own data, consistent with recommendations by the President's Council of Advisors on Science and Technology (2010). However, using this method, matching speed decreases, especially if there are network or participant system delays. In contrast, centralized matching stores all patient identity data centrally, and matching can be done within a single system, avoiding network and provider system delays (Dimitropoulos et al., 2009).

Matching algorithms can employ a blocking scheme to speed the matching process by hierarchically structuring the search for matches. These schemes first block, or group, the data according to one or more fields in the identifying data (e.g., first letter of last name or last digit of SSN) and then carry out the matching process within each block. Records with incorrect data in the blocking field(s) will be put in the wrong group and fail to match when they should, so it is important to select a matching field(s) that has been evaluated and found to be highly accurate. Blocking algorithms using multiple schemes are more accurate and still more efficient than matching algorithms without blocking.

Experiences with Patient Identity Matching for Health Information Technology

None of the research described above assessed patient identity matching outcomes in a functioning HIO with multiple providers. The studies use either simulated or proxy patient indexes and researchers instead of HIO managers to implement the matching algorithms. Thus, the literature provides very limited real-world information upon which to base a choice of patient identifiers, matching algorithm, match criteria, and manual review of the results of automated matching. More research is needed to assess the cost-effectiveness of the different options in practice, using actual patient registries or electronic medical records and the business processes that providers and HIOs are likely to sustain over time.

We were able to gather some information about the VLER experience through our interviews. Like many HIOs, the MHS and the VA currently use SSN, first and last name, date of birth, and gender for patient identity matching in their two systems. They began with a simple deterministic matching algorithm but have been exploring probabilistic algorithms. Although identity matching between the two departments places primary reliance on a unique individual identifier (SSN currently and EDI-PI in the future), a probabilistic matching algorithm will be needed for patients without the identifier and for HIE with civilian providers. Even hospital data systems often lack SSNs for all patients or list the wrong SSNs. Missing and incorrect identifiers will likely limit the ability of VLER to share information with more than a small number of civilian provider organizations for some time.

The MHS, the VA, and civilian providers participating in VLER use NwHIN's CONNECT system to exchange patient information. The matching process is initiated when one provider submits identifying information to CONNECT, which then looks for a match to that information in the other providers' records using a matching algorithm selected for VLER. Both the list of identifiers and the algorithm can differ depending on participants' data availability, data quality, and preferences. When a potential match is identified at another organization, both the requestor and the responding organization must confirm the match for it to be recorded. Multiple matches are treated the same as non-matches, by sending the requester a no-match reply. Until very recently, CONNECT searched for matches one organization at a time, a slow procedure, but it can now perform parallel searches at multiple organizations.

The first VLER site in San Diego, with the VA and Kaiser Permanente as the active participants, planned to use a longer list of identifiers (adding middle initial or name, marital status, address, and phone number) and the deterministic matching algorithm to match patient identity (Bouhaddou et al., 2011). Based on a manual review of 100 patients, only 4 percent of patients were expected to match on all variables. Dropping all of the extra identifiers except address and cleaning discrepancies in the data where possible raised the expected match rate to 50 percent. Cleaning efforts continued to support a match for all patients who were known to have sought care in both systems and who had consented to HIE. A probabilistic algorithm (not described by Bouhaddou et al.) has replaced the original deterministic algorithm, and both organizations have adopted HL7 (Health Level Seven International) data standards to ensure that the identifying variables are recorded the same way in their systems.

The experiences at other VLER sites have not been formally evaluated in the same way that the San Diego experience has. Through our interviews, we learned that the MTFs' experience in patient matching at the sites has been limited. The MTFs have received lists of their patients with information available through VLER and have developed local approaches to retrieving the information and making it available to providers. Few patients had VLER information, and MTF providers found VLER of limited use, since it does not include many civilian providers or provide information for family members.[8] The sites also consistently described slow response times for retrieving patient information, even at this low volume. Interviewees indicated that adoption by MTF providers would be limited unless information was routinely and quickly available for all their patients getting care elsewhere.

Neither the MTF interviewees nor the individuals at higher levels in the MHS we talked to were able to provide information about the accuracy of the patient matching approach (e.g., false negatives, false positives). Several interviewees brought up concerns about duplicate beneficiary enrollment records. DMDC has made efforts to clear duplicate records from its PDR, but new duplicates continue to be generated when patients seek care from an MTF, particularly for patients whose information is not stored locally. Revising MTF work processes to ensure that MTF personnel check the central repository before generating a new patient record and, in the future, checking patients in by swiping their ID cards should cut down substantially on the generation of duplicates. TMA has also had a project to correct inconsistencies in patient identifiers in the various health IT systems and expects that swiping patient ID cards will decrease the problem in the future.

To inform the development of procedures for identity matching in VLER with civilian providers, DMDC ran a test to estimate the number of individuals who would have the same traits if name, birth date, and gender, but not SSN, were used for matching. With an estimated 35 million records (roughly the total population eligible for DoD and VA benefits), there would be 4,000 people who share the same traits. For this reason, and because match rates with civilian providers appear to be low without substantial manual effort, DoD requires civilian providers to use SSN to match patients through VLER. Inter-

---

[8]   Initially, the information provided was limited; patient care summaries became available only later.

viewees who have been most involved in identity matching in VLER all indicated that a national patient identifier will be needed for HIE to function on a national scale.

The VLER pilot did not involve more than a minimal level of information exchange with civilian providers at a few sites. Our interviews revealed a strong interest in expanding VLER to include family members. They emphasized the importance of HIE with civilian providers since they provide over half the services delivered to TRICARE patients overall and specialty care for many of the patients managed by MTFs. As more civilian providers acquire health IT systems capable of supporting HIE and meeting meaningful use requirements, it will be important to systematically identify issues in matching identities between VLER and systems not specifically designed for TRICARE patients. The systems will need to support matching using the identifiers TRICARE designates, and the providers will need to ensure that identifiers in their systems are accurate and the right patient matches are made. The civilian network has over 325,000 providers. Identity management is only one of the significant challenges the MHS will face in expanding HIE to include them.

Summary

Without a national system of unique patient identifiers, patient identity matching for HIE poses difficult challenges. Even if a unique patient identifier were to be established, errors in recording it would require matching on other patient identifiers to ensure that the right patient's information is being exchanged. Considering the different combinations of patient identifiers that are potentially available and the many algorithms that can be adapted to this use, the number of patient identity matching approaches is very large. Unfortunately, there is very limited information available to guide the choice of approach.

As with patient consent, DoD and the VA could inform their own choices and contribute valuable information to guide others by investigating the performance of promising approaches for patient identity management to support nationwide implementation of VLER for all beneficiaries, including military family members and an increasing number of civilian providers. In the concluding chapter of this report, we identify specific topics for research needed to support HIE for military patients.

CHAPTER FIVE

Conclusions and Recommendations

Successful HIE depends on critical mass. Without widespread adoption of EHRs and the supporting infrastructure, HIE cannot be successful. Although DoD has been at the forefront of health IT adoption, uptake among civilian providers in the United States has been relatively slow and uneven—as evident most recently in revisions and extensions to meaningful use criteria and in the general lack of success in RHIOs. To achieve nationwide implementation of VLER for all beneficiaries, including military family members, the primary challenges for the MHS to address pertain to data exchange with civilian providers.

Below we review gaps in research, policy, and practice that need to be addressed to bring about improved quality and efficiency of care through HIE, particularly to support the exchange of health information in the MHS. We describe these issues in terms of the sociotechnical framework adapted from the IOM and provide recommendations for future research. A summary of these issues and recommendations is shown in Table 5.1.

Patient Consent

The predominant technical challenge with respect to patient consent is recording patients' preferences and designing procedures to implement restrictions on disclosures of PHI. Retaining PHI from non-DoD providers (consistent with future plans for VLER) will also require implementing any restrictions on secondary disclosure—a particularly

Table 5.1
Issues and Gaps in Patient Identity Matching and Consent

Factor	Patient Consent	Patient Identity Matching

Technical	1. Data segmentation
	  • Methods
	  • Accommodating preferences
	2. Secondary disclosure
	3. Architecture for patient consent management service
	  • Design
	  • Patient uptake
		1. Performance of matching algorithms
		  • Use actual data
		  • At scale
		2. Pilot in clinical settings

People	1. Provide patient outreach/education
	2. Train clinical and administrative staff
	  • To administer informed consent
	  • To ensure valid, informed consent
	3. Understand patient attitudes and skills with respect to a consent management service
		1. Determine expertise needed for development and maintenance of matching approach(es)
		2. Train clinical and administrative staff on new work processes
		3. Educate beneficiaries about patient matching procedures
		4. Methods for inducing patients to update personal information

Process	1. Analyze/design work processes
	  • To administer informed consent
	  • To verify consent to use and disclose data
		1. Analyze work processes needed for accurate patient identifying data in the PDR
		2. Analyze/design administrative and clinical work processes needed for efficient retrieval and verification of data exchanged electronically

Organization	1. Policy for meaningful, revocable consent 2. Effectiveness of opt-in and opt-out models 3. Governance—involvement of stakeholders in policy development	1. Determine resources needed for development and maintenance of matching approach(es) 2. Policy regarding identifiers for matching with civilian providers
Environment	1. Policy for consent for HIE across states 2. Development of patient-centered consent portal	1. Federal and state policy, e.g., national patient identifier 2. Future development of NwHIN

thorny topic that has received little attention in the literature. Thus, research is needed on the design and usability of automated text processing, particularly with respect to segmenting PHI based on the content of information.

As noted in Chapter Four, we anticipate that national implementation of VLER will require a meaningful consent procedure. To be meaningful, the consent procedure must adequately inform patients about the choices they have, including the opportunity to restrict disclosure, and the consequences of each choice. The procedure must also be conducted in a manner that ensures the consent is understood and is voluntary. As the Tiger Team has pointed out, presenting a consent form without understandable explanation at the moment the patient needs care is not a meaningful consent procedure. The MAeHC has shown that high rates of opt-in consent are feasible but require a well-designed process and considerable outreach. If DoD determines that there should be some kind of consent for HIE through VLER, research addressing people, process, and organizational issues is needed to guide decisions about the type of consent, beneficiary outreach and education, and procedure(s) to be followed to administer and verify consent for HIE at the point of care. Development of such a consent policy would benefit from a governance structure that involves diverse stakeholders, including patients.

Furthermore, the Tiger Team concluded that presentation of the consent protocol by the provider is important to instill trust in HIE. Research on work processes should address how presentation of the consent procedure affects clinical workflows.

We also suggested that development of a patient consent management system for non–active duty beneficiaries may be the best option to meet consent requirements, including the HIPAA requirement for an opt-out procedure and the requirements of civilian providers. Although various architectures for consent management services have been developed, there are few studies of these systems. Pilot tests of these systems in clinical settings are needed to assess their uptake by patients and overall effectiveness.

There are also broader policy issues to address regarding consent for HIE. Most relevant to VLER are (1) challenges in reconciling conflicts among consent requirements across states and between state and federal law and (2) whether patients prefer to use a single portal to manage their consent for all providers and health plans.

Patient Identity Matching

Primary gaps in research on patient identity matching include knowledge regarding the best technical approaches to performing matches and how best to monitor results over time. Research should evaluate the match performance of different approaches involving different combinations of identifiers and algorithms. Moreover, studies should be conducted at the scale that will be required for VLER at the national level once more civilian providers participate in NwHIN. The research should use actual identifying data from the PDR, test performance at scale, and pilot promising approaches in the clinical setting. This work should measure the trade-offs among key performance outcomes, i.e., false negative and false positive rates. Whereas it is relatively straightforward to measure false positive rates by evaluating "hits," it is much more difficult to evaluate false negatives. In addition, research is needed to determine ways to monitor performance over time and should include a focus on the related people, process, and organizational issues, e.g., the expertise and resources needed for development and maintenance of the matching approach.

A parallel line of research should focus on broader people, process, and organizational issues related to the implementation of patient identity matching procedures. Principal outcome measures of these studies would include the speed and accuracy of the patient identity matching approach and how those outcomes affect the providers' uptake of HIE capability and their use of data obtained through HIE in their clinical practice. This research should investigate the following:

- work processes at the facility and system levels within the MHS and the VHA for ensuring the accuracy of patient identifying information in the PDR

- clinical processes and needed changes in clinical and administrative workflows for efficient retrieval and verification of electronic information from other providers to support patient care
- training for clinical and administrative staff
- best practices in outreach and education for beneficiaries about the identity matching procedures to build trust in VLER and engage patients in identifying inaccurate information
- identity management challenges as more civilian providers participate in VLER.

Finally, there are policy issues to resolve within organizations and, in the external environment, at the federal and state levels regarding (1) the types of identifiers that can maintain patient privacy and (2) the further development of NwHIN to support HIE at the scale required for nationwide implementation of VLER for all TRICARE beneficiaries and providers.

Broader Considerations

Finally, it is important to consider how these factors work together to support HIE. In their evaluation of the summary care record in England, Greenhalgh et al. (2010) found that delays in technical solutions, in combination with challenges in obtaining sufficient resources, engaging and training users, aligning work processes, and communicating the change to patients resulted in a protracted implementation process and concomitant loss of motivation. Low uptake of the system was attributed to a number factors in addition to low motivation, including a lack of an integrated technical solution, resulting in the need to log in to multiple systems; insufficient numbers and poor placement of computers, resulting in limited access during office visits; a lack of critical mass; and a lack of management support for its use. Likewise, addressing isolated issues regarding patient consent and identity management will not be productive; research and implementation needs to address multiple factors and their interactions to support successful HIE.

In conclusion, health IT interoperability to support HIE is an important component of the MHS strategic plan. Patient consent and patient identity management are two aspects of HIE that need to be addressed to meet this goal. Achieving interoperability in any context is difficult, but the MHS faces particular challenges related to the ranges of care settings, patient populations, and types of providers involved. Research that addresses patient consent and identity management in the MHS, along with consideration of the underlying privacy issues, will benefit both MHS and the national community of health care stakeholders.

References

Acquisti, Alessandro, and Ralph Gross, "Predicting Social Security Numbers from Public Data," *Proceedings of the National Academy of Sciences,* Vol. 106, No. 27, 2009, pp. 10975–10980.

Adler-Milstein, J., D. W. Bates, and A. K. Jha, "Survey of Health Information Exchange Organizations in the United States: Implications for Meaningful Use," *Annals Internal Medicine,* Vol. 154, 2011, pp. 666–671.

Bouhaddou, Omar, Jamie Bennett, Tim Cromwell, Graham Nixon, Jennifer Teal, Mike Davis, Robert Smith, Linda Fischetti, David Parker, Zachary Gillen, and John Mattison, "The Department of Veterans Affairs, Department of Defense, and Kaiser Permanente Nationwide Health Information Network Exchange in San Diego: Patient Selection, Consent, and Identity Matching," *AMIA Annual Symposium Proceedings,* October 22, 2011, pp. 135–143.

California HealthCare Foundation, *Achieving the Right Balance: Privacy and Security Policies to Support Electronic Health Information Exchange,* June 2011. As of June 13, 2012:
http://www.chcf.org/publications/2012/06/achieving-right-balance

Chow, Richard, Phillippe Golle, and Jessica Staddon, "Detecting Privacy Leaks Using Corpus-Based Association Rules," paper presented at 14th ACM SIGKDD International Conference on Knowledge Discovery and Data Mining, Las Vegas, Nev., August 24–27, 2008.

Creekmore, Rob, John Piescik, and Nahum Gershon, *Megachange Profiler How-to Guide,* McLean, Va.: MITRE, October 2010.

Davis, Fred D., Richard P. Bagozzi, and Paul R. Warshaw, "User Acceptance of Computer Technology: A Comparison of Two Theoretical Models," *Management Science,* Vol. 35, 1989, pp. 982–1003.

del Carmen, Marcela G., and Steven Joffe, "Informed Consent for Medical Treatment and Research: A Review," *The Oncologist,* Vol. 10, 2005, pp. 636–641.

Department of Defense and Department of Veterans Affairs, "Virtual Lifetime Electronic Record (VLER) Initiative: 2010–2014 Strategic Plan V. 2.0," April 8, 2011.

Dimitropoulos, Linda L., Shaun J. Grannis, Alison K. Banger, and David H. Harris, *Privacy and Security Solutions for Interoperable Health Information Exchange*, Chicago: RTI International, June 30, 2009.

Dimitropoulos, Linda, Vaishali Patel, Scott A. Scheffler, and Steve Posnack, "Public Attitudes Toward Health Information Exchange: Perceived Benefits and Concerns," *American Journal of Managed Care,* Vol. 17, December 2011, pp. SP111–SP116.

Dimitropoulos, Linda, and Stephanie Rizk, "A State-Based Approach to Privacy and Security for Interoperable Health Information Exchange," *Health Affairs,* Vol. 28, No. 2, August 2009, pp. 428–434.

Durham, Elizabeth, Yuan Xue, Murat Kantarcioglu, and Bradley Malin, "Private Medical Record Linkage with Approximate Matching," *AMIA Annual Symposium Proceedings*, 2010, pp. 182–186.

eHealth Initiative, "2011 Report on Health Information Exchange: The Changing Landscape," 2011.

Faden, Ruth R., and Tom L. Beauchamp, *A History and Theory of Informed Consent*, New York: Oxford University Press, 1986.

"Federal Register," Vol. 76, November 2, 2011, pp. 67802–67990.

"Federal Register," Vol. 65, No. 250, December 28, 2000.

Ferranti, J. M., R. C. Musser, K. Kawamoto, and W. E. Hammond, "The Clinical Document Architecture and the Continuity of Care Record: A Critical Analysis," *Journal of the American Medical Informatics Association,* Vol. 13, No. 3, 2006, pp. 245–252.

Goldstein, Melissa M., and Alison L. Rein, *Consumer Consent Options for Electronic Health Information Exchange: Policy Considerations and Analysis*, March 23, 2010a.

———, *Data Segmentation in Electronic Health Information Exchange: Policy Considerations and Analysis*, September 29, 2010b.

Grannis, Shaun J., J. Marc Overhage, and Clement J. McDonald, "Analysis of Identifier Performance Using a Deterministic Linkage Algorithm," *AMIA Annual Symposium Proceedings*, 2002, pp. 305–309.

Greenberg, Michael D., and M. Susan Ridgely, *Journal of Health and Biomedical Law,* Vol. 4, No. 1, 2008, pp. 31–68.

Greenberg, Michael D., M. Susan Ridgely, and Richard J. Hillestad, "Crossed Wires: How Yesterday's Privacy Rules Might Undercut Tomorrow's Nationwide Health Information Network," *Health Affairs,* Vol. 29, No. 2, 2009.

Greenhalgh, Trisha, Katja Stramer, Tanja Bratan, Emma Byrne, Jill Russell, and Henry W. W. Potts, "Adoption and Non-Adoption of a Shared Electronic Summary Record in England: A Mixed-Method Case Study," *British Medical Journal,* Vol. 340, 2010, p. c3111.

Greenhalgh, Trisha, Gary W. Wood, Tanja Bratan, Katja Stramer, and Susan Hinder, "Patients' Attitudes to the Summary Care Record and Healthspace: Qualitative Study," *British Medical Journal,* Vol. 336, June 7, 2008, pp. 1290–1295.

Halamka, John, "Meaningful Consent," *The Health Care Blog,* 2012.

Hazlehurst, B., H. R. Frost, et al., "Mediclass: A System for Detecting and Classifying Encounter-Based Clinical Events in Any Electronic Medical Record," *Journal of the American Medical Informatics Association,* Vol. 12, No. 5, 2005, pp. 517–529.

Health Research Institute, *Old Data Learns New Tricks: Managing Patient Privacy and Security on a New Data-Sharing Playground*: PricewaterhouseCoopers LLC, September 2011.

Heinze, Oliver, Markus Birkle, Lennart Köster, and Björn Bergh, "Architecture of a Consent Management Suite and Integration into Ihe-Based Regional Health Information Networks," *BMC Medical Informatics and Decision Making,* Vol. 11, No. 58, 2011.

Hillestad, Richard, James H. Bigelow, Basit Chaudhry, Paul Dreyer, Michael D. Greenberg, Robin C. Meili, M. Susan Ridgely, Jeff Rothenberg, and Roger Taylor, *Identity Crisis: An Examination of the Costs and Benefits of a Unique Patient Identifier for the U.S. Health Care System,* Santa Monica, Calif.: RAND Corporation, MG-753-HLTH, 2008. As of October 18, 2012: http://www.rand.org/pubs/monographs/MG753.html

HIMSS, *Electronic Medical Records Vs. Electronic Health Records: Yes, There Is a Difference,* January 26, 2006.

———, *Patient Identity Integrity,* December 2009. As of August 15, 2012: http://www.himss.org/asp/ContentRedirector.asp?ContentID=76274

———, "Common HIE Technical Architecture Models," in *The HIMSS Guide to Participating in a Health Information Exchange,* 2012.

HITSP, *Manage Consent Directives Transaction Package,* HITSP/TP30, July 8, 2009a.

———, *Security and Privacy Technical Note,* HITSP/TN900, July 8, 2009b.

Hsieh, G., "Towards Self-Protecting Security for E-Health CDA Documents," *International Conference on Security & Management,* 2011.

IBM, *Integrating Patient Medical Records in Pursuit of the EMR,* IMW14343-USEN, September 24, 2010.

Institute of Medicine, *Health IT and Patient Safety: Building Safer Systems for Better Care*, Washington, D.C., 2012.

Interagency Program Office: Annual Report to Congress, Department of Defense and Department of Veterans Affairs.

Junghans, Cornelia, Gene Feder, Harry Hemingway, Adam Timmis, and Melvyn Jones, "Recruiting Patients to Medical Research: Double Blind Randomised Trial of 'Opt-In' Versus 'Opt-Out' Strategies," *British Medical Journal*, Vol. 331, No. 7522, October 22, 2005, pp. 940–942.

Mandl, K. D., P. Szolovits, et al., "Public Standards and Patients' Control: How to Keep Electronic Medical Records Accessible but Private," *British Medical Journal*, Vol. 322, 2001, pp. 283–287.

Markle Foundation, *Markle Common Framework*, undated. As of October 18, 2012:
http://www.markle.org/health/markle-common-framework

Markle Foundation, *Markle Survey on Health in a Networked Life 2010*, January 2011. As of June 14, 2012:
http://www.markle.org/publications/1461-public-and-doctors-overwhelmingly-agree-health-it-priorities-improve-patient-care

McGraw, Deven, James X. Dempsey, Leslie Harris, and Janlori Goldman, "Privacy as an Enabler, Not an Impediment: Building Trust into Health Information Exchange," *Health Affairs*, Vol. 28, No. 2, 2009, pp. 416–427.

McGraw, Deven, and Paul Egerman, "Tiger Team Recommendation Letter," to David Blumenthal, Chair, HIT Policy Committee, August 19, 2010.

Military Health System, *MHS IM/IT Strategic Plan: 2010–2015*, 2009. As of August 14, 2012:
http://www.health.mil/MHSCIO/imitstratplan.aspx

Miller, Robert H., "Satisfying Patient-Consumer Principles for Health Information Exchange: Evidence from California Case Studies," *Health Affairs*, Vol. 31, No. 3, March 1, 2012, pp. 537–547.

Mork, P., A. Rosenthal, and J. Stanford, *Architectures and Processes for Nationwide Patient-Centric Consent Management*, 2011. As of July 3, 2012:
http://www.docstoc.com/docs/111112867Nationwide-Patient-Centric-Consent-Mgmt

National Alliance for Health Information Technology, *Defining Key Health Information Technology Terms*, 2008.

Office for Civil Rights, *OCR Privacy Brief: Summary of the HIPAA Privacy Rule*, U.S. Department of Health and Human Services.

Office of the National Coordinator for Health Information Technology, *National Privacy and Security Framework for Electronic Exchange of Individually Identifiable Health Information*, December 15, 2008. As of June 13, 2012:
http://healthit.hhs.gov/portal/server.pt/
communityhealthit_hhs_gov__privacy___security_framework/1173

———, *Nationwide Health Information Network: Overview*, May 20, 2011.

Patel, Vaishali N., Rina V. Dhopeshwarkar, Alison Edwards, Yolanda Barrón, Jeffrey Sparenborg, and Rainu Kaushal, "Consumer Support for Health Information Exchange and Personal Health Records: A Regional Health Information Organization Survey," *Journal of Medical Systems,* Vol. 36, 2012, pp. 36, 1043–1052.

President's Commission on Care for America's Returning Wounded Warriors, "Serve, Support, Simplify," July 2007.

President's Council of Advisors on Science and Technology, *Report to the President: Realizing the Full Potential of Health Information Technology to Improve Healthcare for Americans: The Path Forward*, December 2010. As of June 14, 2012:
http://www.whitehouse.gov/sites/default/files/microsites/ostp/
pcast-health-it-report.pdf

President's Task Force to Improve Health Care Delivery for the Nation's Veterans, *Final Report*, 2003.

Pritts, Joy, and Kathleen Connor, *The Implementation of E-Consent Mechanisms in Three Countries: Canada, England, and the Netherlands,* Health Policy Institute, Georgetown University, February 16, 2007. As of August 14, 2012:
http://ihcrp.georgetown.edu/pdfs/prittse-consent.pdf

Sicotte, Claude, and Guy Paré, "Success in Health Information Exchange Projects: Solving the Implementation Puzzle," *Social Science and Medicine,* Vol. 70, No. 8, April 2010, pp. 1159–1165.

Simon, Steven R., J. Stewart Evans, Alison Benfamin, David Delano, and David W. Bates, "Patients' Attitudes Toward Electronic Health Information Exchange: Qualitative Study," *Journal of Medical Internet Research,* Vol. 11, No. 3, 2009.

Sittig, D. F., and H. Singh, "A New Sociotechnical Model for Studying Health Information Technology in Complex Adaptive Healthcare Systems," *Quality and Safety in Health Care Journal,* Vol. 19, 2007, pp. 68–74.

Skentzos, S., M. Shubina, et al., "Structured Vs. Unstructured: Factors Affecting Adverse Drug Reaction Documentation in an EMR Repository," *American Medical Informatics Association,* 2011.

Staddon, Jessica, Philippe Golle, and Bryce Zimny, "Web-Based Inference Detection," *16th USENIX Security Symposium,* Boston, Mass., August 8, 2007, pp. 71–86.

Stanley, Belinda, Jane Fraser, and N. H. Cox, "Uptake of HIV Screening in Genito-Urinary Medicine After Change to "Opt-Out" Consent," *British Medical Journal,* Vol. 326, May 31, 2003, p. 1174.

TRICARE, *Evaluation of the Tricare Program: Fiscal Year 2012 Report to Congress,* TRICARE Management Activity, February 28, 2012. As of May 15, 2012: http://www.tricare.mil/tma/StudiesEval.aspx

Tripathi, Micky, David Delano, Barbara Lund, and Lynda Rudolph, "Engaging Patients for Health Information Exchange," *Health Affairs,* Vol. 28, No. 2, 2009, pp. 435–443.

Turchin, A., M. Shubina, et al., "Comparison of Information Content of Structured and Narrative Text Data Sources on the Example of Medication Intensification," *Journal of the American Medical Informatics Association,* Vol. 16, No. 3, 2009, pp. 362–370.

Under Secretary of Defense (Personnel and Readiness), "DoD Social Security Number (SSN) Reduction Plan," April 28, 2008.

Unertl, K. M., K. B. Johnson, et al., "Health Information Exchange Technology on the Front Lines of Healthcare: Workflow Factors and Patterns of Use," *Journal of the American Medical Informatics Association,* 2011.

U.S. Department of Veteran's Affairs, *My HealtheVet,* September 24, 2012. As of October 18, 2012: https://www.myhealth.va.gov/

Venkatesh, Viswanath, and Fred D. Davis, "A Theoretical Extension of the Technology Acceptance Model: Four Longitudinal Field Studies," *Management Science,* Vol. 46, No. 2, 2000, pp. 186–204.

Venkatesh, Viswanath, Michael G. Morris, Gordon B. Davis, and Fred D. Davis, "User Acceptance of Information Technology: Toward a Unified View," *MIS Quarterly,* Vol. 27, No. 3, September 2003, pp. 425–478.

West, Darrell M., and Allan Friedman, *Health Information Exchanges and Megachange,* Washington, D.C.: Brookings, February 2012.

Westat, *Consumer Engagement in Developing Electronic Health Information Systems,* AHRQ 09-0081-EF, July 2009.

Wilcox, Adam, Gilad Kuperman, David A. Dorr, George Hripcsak, Scott P. Narus, Sidney N. Thornton, and R. Scott Evans, "Architectural Strategies and Issues with Health Information Exchange," *AMIA Annual Symposium Proceedings,* 2006, pp. 814–818.